Aromatherapy for Women

Aromatherapy for Women

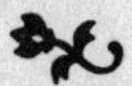

How to use the remarkable beautifying and healing qualities of essential oils

Maggie Tisserand

Thorsons

An Imprint of HarperCollins*Publishers*

Thorsons
An Imprint of HarperCollins*Publishers*
77–85 Fulham Palace Road,
Hammersmith, London W6 8JB

Published by Thorsons 1985, 1990
This revised edition published 1993
13 15 14

A catalogue record for this book
is available from the British Library

ISBN 0 7225 2260 6

Phototypeset by Harper Phototypesetters Limited,
Northampton, England
Printed in Great Britain by
Caledonian International Book Manufacturer, Glasgow

CONTENTS

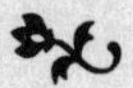

ACKNOWLEDGEMENTS

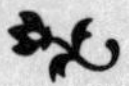

Thanks to my friend Sue Robinson, who helped to edit many of the chapters.

Grateful thanks to my three children for being so trusting in me, and for the opportunities given to me to treat them, even for serious illnesses, and to put my faith to the test.

INTRODUCTION

Firstly, I would like to explain my reasons for the title of my book, and apologize to all those men who have said to me 'What about aromatherapy for men?' Of course, aromatherapy is not only for women: it is for any human being - woman, child or man - and also for animals, in certain circumstances. I chose the title as there is a large proportion of the book relating to pregnancy, childbirth and gynaecological problems, which are only pertinent to women, but there is much information contained in the book which will be of benefit to men, especially the section about 'Aromatherapy and the immune system' (Chapter 6).

For much of the book I have drawn largely on my own experiences during pregnancy, childbirth and in bringing up three children; in the visible improvements in my appearance and the general state of my health; and also on feedback from friends and relatives who have benefited from using essential oils.

In a nutshell, aromatherapy means 'a therapy using aromas'. The aromas come from the plant kingdom - flowers, trees, bushes, and herbs. The relevant part of the plant (the wood of the sandalwood tree; the petals of the rose; the peel of the lemon; the leaves of rosemary bushes; berries of the juniper tree, etc) is put through a process of distillation, where the volatile, odiferous substance is captured. It is this liquid which is known as an essential oil.

Essential oils have many uses, although our sense of smell, being linked to our emotions, plays the largest part in recognizing the power of aromatherapy and it is here that we can discover how certain essences have the power to lift depression, or which essences have a calming influence on troubled emotions. Aromatherapy is a mixture of aromas, massage and medicine.

It was in 1972 that I first looked for an alternative form of medicine, when I decided that I no longer wanted to take aspirins or antibiotics. Homoeopathy was the alternative science that I chose to study, but whilst living in a sort of 'medical commune' with other like-minded young people, something happened which was to imprint itself forever in my memory - the miraculous healing power of essential oils! One day a friend turned up on the doorstep, nursing a badly burned arm. He had removed the radiator cap from his Jeep, and a jet of steam had seared the skin from his forearm. He resolutely refused to go to hospital, insisting that we treat him. Annie (an SRN nurse and trainee acupuncturist) diagnosed the injury as being a second-degree burn, and tidied up the site of injury with sterile instruments. I administered homoeopathic arnica to lessen the shock, and Robert Tisserand applied neat lavender oil on sterile gauze. The essence stung at first, but then reduced the pain, and this treatment was employed twice a day for a little over a week. After two weeks the arm was completely healed, there was no scar tissue, and our friend was able to return to work.

Lavender oil had been chosen because it had been used by Gattefosse in the 1930s and later by Dr Valnet - both in the treatment of burns, and both with remarkable results. Witnessing for myself the incredible healing power of essential oils in this way was the start of a long love affair with aromatherapy.

During my 11-year marriage to Robert Tisserand, now a leading aromatherapist, I literally 'lived and breathed' aromatherapy, utilizing essential oils for health, beauty and well-being, and although I am now divorced from Robert, my love for aromatherapy and my appreciation and respect for essential oils just gets stronger.

The subject of aromatherapy is so complex, yet at the same time so very simple to put into practice, that anyone can embark on the journey of aromatherapy, beginning with an aromatic bath and then, if so inclined, to go on studying aromatherapy for the rest of his or her life. There is always more to learn.

Having confidence is important when treating your family's minor ailments using essential oils. I have confidence to treat my children because of my knowledge of the essences, my intuition, and my trust in the loving power that put the essences into the plants. When we are sick we have to put our trust in someone or something, and that someone can be a doctor, a pharmacist, or yourself, and that something can be a doctor's prescription, an over-the-counter drug, or aromatherapy. The choice is yours.

Throughout this book, I have expressed opinions which may offend some medical personnel. I am not 'anti-doctor'; in fact, several of my friends are doctors, but I strongly oppose the over-use of prescribed drugs. Modern medicine has much to offer, especially with regard to technological life-saving techniques, and if I were ever run over by a bus, I would certainly be thankful for this facility. However, I see nothing to be proud of in the way that our hospitals are used as an outlet for the drug companies' products, costing the National Health Service millions of pounds per year, when cheaper, more effective, and more user-friendly remedies are available. A few hospitals in the UK are now incorporating aromatherapy into their patient care, with quite astounding results (in one Oxford hospital ward the administration of night-time sedatives has been significantly reduced as patients are offered an aromatherapy massage instead, and some wards are using essential oils on burners to purify the atmosphere); however, the use of essential oils in hospitals is still only employed on a very small scale. A recent report outlines the dangers of picking up infections whilst in hospital, and according to this report, the longer your stay in hospital, the more likely you are to acquire an infection which could prolong your hospital stay. This reinforces my observations and comments about maternity hospitals being dangerous places for babies and for the newly-delivered mother, and emphasizes the need to take our 'healthy atmosphere' with us. By surrounding ourselves with the protective aromas of plants, we can prevent the likelihood of succumbing to airborne bacteria. Aromatherapy is not just to treat an illness which has developed, but is a very real protection from environmental pollutants, bacteria and viruses. Instead of waiting for the body to manifest the pathological changes of disease, we have the tools available to protect the body and to build up resistance to disease, so that ill-health does not occur. We are at the beginning of a health revolution. Preventive medicine is the medicine of the future, and aromatherapy is one of the important therapies of the 1990s.

By keeping ourselves healthy and functioning efficiently, we automatically pay fewer visits to our doctor, thereby freeing him or her from the humdrum and repetitive prescribing of non-essential medicines, and allowing his or her skills to be channelled to the very sick and dying patient.

The reason for taking a trivial complaint to a doctor can no longer be excused in terms of 'well it's free - I have already paid for the NHS in my taxes'. Now that each prescription charge is several pounds in value, it is possible to purchase a bottle of essential oil for almost the same price. As nearly all essential oils have excellent 'keeping qualities', every time we buy an essential oil, unlike the 'course' of prescribed drugs which must be finished or thrown away, we are investing in long-term health by building up a collection of potent plant medicines. Furthermore, by utilising plant oils for our health needs, our bodies are no longer excreting antibiotics and other harmful drugs into the sea, via the sewage system. Aromatherapy is a truly holistic therapy, not only for humans but also for the planet.

Aromatherapy is very important to me, and my knowledge of aromatherapy has been the best investment, in terms of health and beauty, that I have ever made. I hope that by sharing my experiences with you, opinionated as they may seem, you will find in aromatherapy a valuable adjunct to other forms of alternative medicine and a very practical, highly enjoyable way of feeling and looking good.

Chapter One

GETTING THROUGH THE DAY

DEPRESSION

A big black cloud, blotting out the light from the sun, is how I describe depression when it happens to me. But as depression is something that affects most of us at one time or another, the way in which it manifests itself will vary from one person to another. One friend of mine describes it as like 'wandering through thick fog, not knowing in which direction I am walking, and not knowing when or if the fog will lift'.

Another friend describes depression as being like an invisible, suffocating weight which she has to carry, and which makes her so exhausted that she feels tired all of the time. She told me that when recently depressed, and lying on her bed in the middle of the day thinking about her dire financial problems and wallowing in self-pity, a thought came into her head 'like a distress flare at sea', to turn to aromatherapy for help. Knowing that certain essences are beneficial in lifting depression she got up off the bed, sorted through her oil collection, and put three drops of **clary sage** onto her fragrancer, closed the door and window and again lay down on her bed, thinking that although she was beyond help, she ought to give it a try. This is how she described the following half hour:

> 'It was incredible. Within minutes I was feeling lighter. I began to feel happier and less worried. The money problem was still there, but somehow I felt detached from it, as though it had been put into a balloon, which was floating above my

> head even though it was still attached to me by a string. The stifling weight which had robbed me of my energy and inner harmony was not there any more, and after 30 minutes I felt like getting up and getting on with things.

She experienced more energy than she had had for several days, and began to function normally again. Contrast this with the stories of women who have become addicted to tranquillizers, having been prescribed them for depression.

Some people find **clary sage** to be euphoric, and will not use the essence in their working environment for fear of becoming too light-headed. I like to use **clary sage** in my office occasionally, possibly because I don't really like paper work, and doing it makes me feel moody. I have a theory about **clary sage**. Imagine that our emotions are like an elevator or lift, and that our normal state is the ground floor; when depressed we travel down to the lower ground floor, and when euphoric, we are on the first floor. Imagine that **clary sage** has the ability to take us up one floor level. If we are depressed, it returns us to the ground floor, but if we are already normal then it takes us to the first floor. This would explain why different people have different experiences with this essence. But the common denominator is that **clary sage** is emotionally uplifting.

Jet-Lag

My three children arrived back from a two-week stay in Michigan absolutely exhausted. It was their first transatlantic flight since they were babies, so they were not at all 'seasoned travellers'. On arriving home at 10 in the morning after an 11-hour journey, they each had a bowl of cereal and went to bed. I wasn't sure whether to wake them up later in the day, or let them continue to sleep in the vain hope that they might sleep for 24 hours. Unfortunately they only managed 14 hours, which meant that by midnight they were wide awake and remained so until 6.30 the following morning. I did not want the strange sleeping pattern to continue for too long, so I woke them up at midday. To say that they were tired would be an understatement, so each had a bath with **rosemary** and **geranium** oils, after which their vitality seemed to be increased.

Over the next few hours they all seemed to be in a depressive, lethargic state, and so I decided to conduct an experiment. I sent one child off to bed for an hour's nap, as a 'control'. One daughter had dilute **rose** oil rubbed onto her neck, hands and wrist. My third child (who had been the most grumpy) was given some oils to smell. I put drops of **jasmine, lemon** and **bergamot** oils onto a tissue and wafted this under his nose. Of course he protested, saying that it was horrible, but the reaction was remarkable. Within two minutes he smiled and said 'I feel better already.' Every so often he would shiver slightly, as if he were very cold, and described these sensations as being like ripples going through his muscles. It seemed to me that his body was letting go of the stress and tension encountered by most air travellers. His sleep patterns returned to normal much faster than that of his sisters, who needed a nightly massage to get them off to sleep.

I have my own way of coping with jet-lag; I don't allow myself to have it. When flying back from the west coast of America, I try to get a flight which arrives mid-morning UK-time. This means that I can drive home and be in bed by about 1 p.m., having set my alarm for 6 p.m. Sometimes it seems hard, but at 6 p.m. I force myself out of bed, and into a **rosemary** and **geranium** bath. Then I go to the supermarket to re-stock my groceries, followed by a light meal in a restaurant. Ten o'clock is when I allow myself to go to bed, and just to make sure that I have a deep sleep, I unplug the phones and put some **marjoram** oil onto a tissue or on the ceramic burner. Next morning, at about 9 a.m., I get up, have another **rosemary** and **lemongrass** bath, and tell myself that it's just a normal day. Then I just go ahead and have a normal day (although I can't handle anything which requires mental dexterity). As long as I continue the morning **rosemary** baths, and make sure I am in bed by 10 p.m. then I find that my body rhythms very quickly become readjusted, and I can truthfully say that I do not suffer from jet-lag.

Travel Sickness

When my children were younger travel sickness was something I tried hard to guard against, because vomit is one aroma which I am not partial to! My eldest daughter would often complain of feeling sick while travelling on motorways. If she had been eating I would give her **peppermint** oil to smell, as **peppermint** is renowned for its stomachic properties (calming the stomach). Nervous tension is also a cause of travel sickness, and in this case the aroma of **lavender** would be more beneficial, as it is soothing and calming. The easiest way to use these essences without fear of spillage is to put one drop of either **peppermint** or **lavender** onto a tissue, and breathe in the vapours. Only on one occasion have I needed to clean up the back seat of my car, and then it was my fault for allowing my daughter to eat a huge cream-cake in a motorway service station. If a child (or adult for that matter) is prone to feeling car sick, the choice of foods taken before and during travel should be given careful consideration.

Lavender and **peppermint** oil on a tissue is the easiest way of breathing in the soothing vapours. A tissue impregnated with these oils can be placed inside a small plastic bag (sandwich-bag-sized) and popped into the glove compartment. When needed, just tear open a small hole in the bag and inhale.

Traveller's Fatigue

Adults often have difficulty in sleeping during a long journey, even though they may be completely exhausted, but at least adults can rationalize that they have a sleep problem, and either read a book, watch the scenery or start up a conversation with a fellow passenger. Not so for a young baby or small child. Rational thinking is beyond them, and so their frustration and anger will manifest itself in crying and screaming. Once, whilst travelling by air to San Francisco, I experienced the desperate frustration of a child who could not get to sleep. The little girl was just over one year old, and very cute. For the first four hours she crawled around and played quite happily, until she was too tired to play any more; then the grizzling started. This turned to progressively louder cries until the mother administered a dose of Fenergen (a proprietary sedative for babies). The Fenergen did not send the child to sleep, but merely induced a sort of a 'high' which lasted for an hour. Then the screaming started. If you have ever been on a plane with a screaming child you know how it feels. You can't go out for a walk. There is nowhere to go to escape the noise, and sleep is impossible. I'm rather shy, but when I could not bear to see and hear the distress any longer, I offered to hold the child for a while to give the mother a break. Prior to doing this, I rubbed some **lavender** oil down the sides of my neck. Walking up and down the galley with a beautiful baby girl in my arms reminded me of the time when my own children were babies, and how incredible babies are. Less than five minutes had gone by before the child was fast asleep and, much to the surprise of the parents, I was able to lay her down in the carrycot, where she slept peacefully until awoken by an air stewardess on our approach to San Francisco airport.

MENTAL FATIGUE

Several oils are mentally stimulating, but I have not found one which surpasses **basil** oil. A drop or two of **basil** on a source of heat such as a bowl of hot water, or specially designed fragrancer is, for me, as good as going for a walk along the sea front. Not only do I feel mentally alert, but refreshed also. I would recommend that office workers keep a bottle of basil in their desk for use mid-afternoon, when 5 o'clock seems so far away; or when the job demands that you work overtime, but your brain doesn't quite feel able to cope.

I have often thought - on reading newspaper reports about overworked hospital doctors struggling to keep awake - that if only they could have a whiff of **basil** oil, it would perk up their brain cells just as coffee does, but without causing any strain on the kidneys.

Other oils which are stimulating and are perfect to use in any situation where tiredness is becoming a problem, whether in the workplace, home or car, are: **rosemary, rosewood, lemongrass** and the citrus oils - **lemon, orange, bergamot** and **grapefruit**.

Basil oil came to my rescue quite by accident one day. Taking my youngest child with me, I decided to drive to Paris to collect her sister who had been staying with friends. We arrived in Calais at dusk, and decided to stay the night, rather than try to drive on the 'wrong' side of the road while tired. I checked in to a nice-looking hotel overlooking a quiet square, but had not realized that the quiet square was going to turn into a noisy fairground at precisely the moment we wanted to take an early night. The loud music and shrieks of the happy customers continued until 2 o'clock in the morning, when I was finally able to go to sleep. This was not for long though, as the dustmen (garbage collectors) arrived before dawn, and made so much noise that I gave up trying to sleep. I decided to have a **rosemary** bath, as I usually do when I need revitalizing, but finding that I had forgotten my **rosemary** oil, I settled for a **basil** bath. **Basil** must be used with caution, as the ingredient which makes it a brain stimulant can also be irritating to the skin. I used just two drops to a full bath, and mixed it thoroughly. I got into the bath feeling absolutely wretched, and convinced that I would never be able to negotiate my way out of Calais, let alone navigate around the Périphérique and find my way to a remote town on the outskirts of Paris. However, half an hour later, I stepped out of the bath feeling as though I could happily undertake Le Mans!

When Children Can't Sleep

Lavender is widely accepted as being a sedative, and is a great help when someone has a difficult time in getting off to sleep.

I have used **lavender** in many ways when my children have complained about not being able to sleep. Sometimes I have given them a **lavender** bath, but this is not always convenient. Sometimes a drop of **lavender** on the edge of the pillow, sometimes on a tissue. Recently I invented a '**lavender** tube', which works better than anything else. When the essence is dropped onto a tissue, it evaporates straight up into the atmosphere, but with a **lavender** tube, the vapour is trapped, and forced out at the end only. I take a sheet of kitchen towel (one of the stiffer types of paper) and put one or two drops of **lavender** on one edge. I then roll the paper into a sausage shape with the **lavender** in the middle. The tube can then be held in the hand by the child, without the essence coming into contact with the skin, and when the child falls asleep, the tube automatically falls from the hand. My daughters think it's great!

ENVIRONMENTAL FRAGRANCE

Offices and other workplaces can become very stuffy, with the air full of everybody else's smells - aftershave, coffee, strong perfumes, cigarette smoke, photocopier chemicals - and this can contribute to a lack of efficiency as the day wears on. Very often in air-conditioned buildings the windows are sealed shut and it is impossible to open them even though you may be craving for some fresh air, but you can freshen the atmosphere quite considerably by sprinkling a few drops of an essential oil around you. Essential oils give off their aromas that much quicker if they are in contact with heat; if there is no source of heat nearby, the most accessible item to most people would probably be a mug of hot water to drop the oils in. Light citrus oils like **rosewood, lemon** or **bergamot**, and fresh herbal aromas such as **rosemary**, not only scent the atmosphere but bring a freshness and clarity. Because all essential oils have antiseptic properties, their use will also offer you some measure of protection from the airborne bacteria with which we are surrounded. Tests in air-conditioned buildings in which staff suffer recurrent illness and lethargy have shown that the atmosphere can indeed become very unhealthy; this pattern of ill-health caused by a working environment is known as 'sick building syndrome'. A Japanese company is now incorporating aromatic vapours into the air-conditioning systems of offices and banks, and finds that **lemon** oil increases efficiency and reduces error. Until the time when all buildings are so equipped, we can carry our own 'environmental fragrance' in our handbag or briefcase, to use as and when required.

Nervous Diarrhoea

Have you ever had to keep rushing to the loo with an upset stomach just before an important occasion? You know you haven't eaten anything terrible, so it must just be 'nerves'. But how can you stop it from happening? **Geranium** oil is sedative and uplifting at the same time, and is used by doctors in Italy to treat anxiety states. One or two drops of the oil, on brown sugar or in honey water (see page 158), and taken an hour or two prior to the event, will soon bring relief whether you are going for a job interview, preparing dinner for someone important, or receiving an Oscar for 'best supporting actress'. **Neroli** oil, which is also used to treat nervous tension and anxiety states, will soothe and calm the central nervous system when worn as a perfume. When **neroli** oil is diluted in **jojoba**, it will 'keep' for a long time, and is a good standby to have in your handbag for those moments when the butterflies threaten to take over.

Muscular Aches

Physical activity has become more popular, both with men and women, and whether you are a regular exercise freak or a complete beginner, there will be occasions when you may overdo it. This is when every muscle in your legs aches, and walking up a flight of stairs becomes an endurance test. It is at such times that I would recommend a massage of the affected part (calf, thigh, upper arm and so on) to bring relief from pain, and to speed up the repair process.

Athletes and professional sports people always have a massage after their training sessions, but few of us are privileged to have our own personal physiotherapist. With a little confidence and some practical experience, however, we can take care of our minor aches and pains, as well as give comfort to a friend in discomfort.

Massage of the legs should always be in a circular movement, and always upwards towards the heart. The pain experienced in the muscles is caused by a build-up of lactic acid, and by massaging the affected muscle, or groups of muscles, beginning gently and gradually applying more pressure as the pain can be tolerated, the lactic acid is encouraged to disperse.

Massage alone will ease the pain and stiffness, and help to restore suppleness to the limbs, but for an even more effective treatment I would always recommend the addition of essential oils into a base oil, and in the recipe section (Chapter 12) you will find a recipe of **lavender, rosemary** and **juniper** which has been found to be of great help.

ACHING FEET

Women's feet have a lot of weight to carry around, and often are forced into narrow and uncomfortable shoes. But standing on a crowded tube train, or running for a bus seem inappropriate times to be concerned with appearances! Every part of our body has a corresponding reflex zone on the foot, and what happens to our feet can easily have an adverse affect on our well-being. Irritability, nausea, headaches, even migraines can occur by forcing our feet to endure hours of torture and mistreatment.

However, I am as guilty as anyone for following fashion dictates, and the way in which I say 'sorry' to my feet and revive myself quickly is to have a footbath as soon as I reach home. Just ten minutes with your feet in a bowl of water, or sitting on the edge of your bath with your feet in a few inches of water to which you have first added a few drops of oil, will work wonders. Gentle massaging of the many reflex zones of the feet will greatly enhance your recuperation. **Peppermint** in cool water is the perfect footbath for a hot summer's day, whilst **myrtle** or **geranium** are warming and comforting aromas when used in warm water on a wintry day.

Foot Odour

Smelly feet can be embarrassing to their owners as well as unpleasant to other people. The habit of wearing nylon socks inside tightly-laced shoes means men suffer from this problem more than women do. Aromatherapy cannot 'cure' foot odour but the use of certain essential oils can bring about a great improvement. **Cypress** oil is a natural deodorant and can be used in a footbath or diluted into a fatty-oil base and massaged into the feet. A daily footbath is very beneficial, with perhaps the addition of a weekly foot massage.

Unwinding After a Tiring Day

Many things can 'wind us up'. Driving, coping with children, attending to countless customers in shops or banks, commuting on packed trains, or partaking in whatever stressful activity is part of our lifestyle. Cigarettes, alcohol and tranquillizers have become the methods of relaxation employed by people in the Western world. A healthy and safe alternative to these measures is to take an aromatic bath each day. Even if you prefer showering for its speed and economy, think of bathing as a therapy and try to take one or two aromatic baths every week. Just as swimming in a warm sea is mentally and physically therapeutic, so too is lying in a warm bath, doing absolutely nothing except to inhale the vapours as they are released into the air. A few drops of your favourite essential oil (particularly good are **neroli, rosewood, myrtle, geranium** or **lavender**) will soothe and gently ease away the mental and physical tensions of the day. The day's events register as physical tension, which is the reason why we get tight neck muscles, headaches, irritability or insomnia. It may seem easier to reach for an analgesic tablet or tranquillizer, but if we stop to think about the effect that the drug is having on our body on an immediate level, and then think about the possible long-term problems associated with those drugs, we may decide that it is much better to opt for a safe alternative, such as an aromatic bath, even if it takes a little more time and effort. Stress, if allowed to build up over a period of weeks, months or years will eventually lead to a breakdown in health; this could manifest itself in the form of a serious health problem such as cancer, ME, MS or some other disease of our time. Daily letting-go of stress and tension could be and should be as routine as brushing our teeth.

Insomnia

Anyone who has a busy lifestyle which sometimes overburdens him or her with worries and responsibilities, may experience the occasional night when sleep is elusive.

While preparing for my exams at school, many years ago, my sleep patterns became very disturbed due to my constant fear of failure. Once the stressful situation was removed - in my case, after I had received the examination results - I was again able to go to bed and fall asleep.

Nowadays, it is a rare occurrence for me to lie awake at night but such is the power of the mind that when a strong thought pattern has been established, and continues to go round in circles, I find that I have to take practical steps to break the circle. If my problem is that I am thinking negative thoughts about someone who has upset me, or I strongly disagree with a decision over which I have no control, then I reach for pen and paper, and write down my thoughts until I have 'got it off my chest'. I may write a letter to someone who has been causing me to feel very negatively, and in my letter I express myself in a very forthright way, imagining the effect it will have on the recipient as he or she reads it. When I feel satisfied that I have unburdened myself, then I sprinkle some **marjoram** oil onto my electric burner, and with the aromas of sweet herbs floating through my mind, I fall asleep. I always find on those nights when I have used **marjoram**, I sleep deeper than normal. Of course, in the morning, I tear up the letter. I don't need to send it: it is enough that I have written down the destructive thoughts, and rid myself of the unpleasant emotions that were robbing me of my rest.

Many people suffer from chronic insomnia, and find that their body's natural rhythms have been so disturbed that the only way in which to fall asleep is to take a nightly tranquillizing drug. It is possible to substitute essential oils for tranquillizers, and to enjoy a good night's sleep without feeling 'hung over' the next morning. **Lavender** is a very strong sedative which, when used in a night-time bath, dissolves away mental and physical tension, and induces a restful night's sleep. Add five or six drops of **lavender** to a comfortably hot bath. Don't wash and scrub - this bath is not for cleanliness but for rest and relaxation - just lie back and wallow; and don't set a time limit on yourself - stay as long as you feel comfortable, adding more hot water as necessary. Some relatives of mine of retirement age swear by their **lavender** baths to help them to sleep at night. Because of the deep sleep they enjoy at night, they are full of vitality during the day.

Common sense must play a part in treating insomnia, and eating the main meal of the day at lunchtime, instead of in the evening, may help considerably. Foods which are known stimulants should be avoided, such as coffee and chocolate, as they could aggravate the inability to 'switch off'. For any insomniac who does not like the aroma of **lavender** or **marjoram**, then a completely different type of aroma is **neroli** (orange blossom). Although very light and floral, **neroli** is still very sedative, and may be used alone or in combination with either **lavender** or **marjoram**. All of these oils can be used in the bath, on the edge of the pillow or in a room fragrancer.

Waking Up at Night

Sometimes the day's events or a particular worry are so strongly entrenched in our minds that even when asleep, the slightest provocation (a cat fight in the garden, or a car door slamming) can awaken us, and it becomes impossible to go back to sleep again. A glance at the clock may tell us that 3 a.m. is far too early to get up, but the mind is chattering away as though it was the middle of the day. This has happened to me on occasions, especially when staying in hotels where everything is unfamiliar (and sometimes uncomfortable). I write down any thoughts that are going through my mind, and then put some **lavender** or **marjoram** oil on a tissue, place the tissue across my face and breathe in the aromatic vapours until sleep comes.

Revitalize Before a Night Out

Occasionally our energy levels can be so depleted at the end of a busy day that there seems to be no enthusiasm to go out socially and enjoy oneself. Sometimes it feels as though you are a car with a flat battery, and without some sort of a boost, there is no way that the car will start. At times like these a half-hour aromatic bath could be just the boost you need. One or two drops of oil, in any of these combinations, will help to revitalize you for the evening ahead; **rosemary** and **rosewood**; **rosemary** and **geranium**; **rosewood** and **bergamot**; or whichever essence you find to be beneficial. If exhaustion has depressed your emotions slightly, then add a drop or two of **clary sage** oil to your bath water. Alternatively, a drop or two of **clary sage** oil may be taken internally, on a little brown sugar or in honey water.

Hangover

Most adults have, at some time or another, experienced a hangover: that unique combination of heavy head, unbelievable pain, nausea, sensitivity to noise and light, and generally feeling like death. This is hardly surprising when you consider that alcohol is actually a poison when taken in excess, disturbing the body chemistry and robbing it of vital fluids. According to one scientist, for every glass of whisky we drink, 1 million brain cells are killed; and if alcohol were invented today, it would never pass the government safety tests on new products.

Nobody ever wants a hangover, but we all overindulge occasionally, and need to recover. Firstly drink a large glass of water, preferably still, bottled water, as alcohol causes dehydration which in turn gives rise to severe headaches. Follow this by a long aromatic bath with **rosemary** or **juniper** (see recipe section). To combat nausea there is nothing finer than a drop of **peppermint** in warm honey water. **Peppermint** can also be taken on a little brown sugar, but I find that hot water increases the speed at which the essential oils reach the bloodstream. If you do not have access to a bath, then you should massage a little **lavender** oil into the nape of the neck and lie down with a **lavender** or **geranium** compress across your forehead. **Jojoba** oil is virtually indigestible, and will coat the lining of the stomach. A teaspoonful taken before going out drinking, may slow down the rate of absorption of the alcohol, but will also interfere with digestion of food, and is only a temporary measure. I still prefer to 'mix' my drinks; one glass of wine or other alcohol, followed by one glass of water.

On occasions I have drunk too much alcohol, as I have a very low tolerance level, and find that the following day I have a dull ache in the middle of my back, as alcohol adversely affects the kidneys. By rubbing **sandalwood** oil (which is extraordinarily good for helping with kidney problems) into this area, I always find that the ache is soothed away, which means that I can get on with the business of the day without discomfort.

Aromatic Teas

Flavoured teas make a welcome alternative to the taste of black tea, and for a while I was a regular user of Earl Grey tea until I became bored with it. As this is just tea flavoured with essential oil of **bergamot** there is no reason why you cannot make your own aromatic teas with essential oils that you have in your collection. Next to **bergamot**, the most obvious choice of oil for a tea would be **peppermint**. You can make your own Earl Grey tea by adding one drop of **bergamot** oil to tea in a pot and adding 3-4 cups of hot water. Either Japanese green tea or Indian black tea may be used, but some essential oils work better with green tea and others with black tea. Black tea should be used with **peppermint** and **bergamot**. Put tea into a pot, add one drop of oil and then add

3-4 cups of hot water. Drink while fresh.

Lemon and **orange** oil may be added to either type of tea and make a delightfully refreshing tea any time of the day; to a teapot add tea, one drop of oil and 1-2 cups of hot water. **Jasmine** oil makes such a wonderful tea that I have put it in the chapter on sex and sexuality (Chapter 3)!

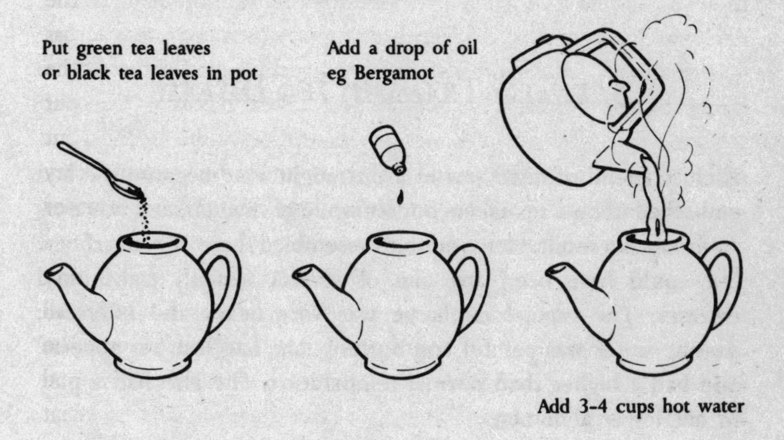

How to make tea with your essential oils

Chapter Two

GYNAECOLOGICAL REMEDIES

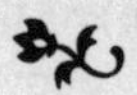

SEXUALLY TRANSMITTED DISEASE

A close friend of mine was in a distraught state because she had embarked upon a sexual encounter while on holiday, and was now suffering as a result. Her symptoms resembled those of gonorrhoea, but could have been any one of several sexually transmitted diseases. The vaginal discharge was very heavy and offensive; passing water was painful and burning; she had lost her appetite and had a higher than normal temperature. She also had a pain in her lower abdomen.

She was feeling so ill and so ashamed of herself that she stayed in bed, and asked me for my help until she felt like going out to the STD clinic. Not knowing what was wrong with her, but knowing that **sandalwood** oil is used in India for the treatment of gonorrhoea (and that it is completely harmless when taken orally), I recommended that she take 6 drops of pure **sandalwood** each day, until she was able to have a diagnosis at the clinic. Time passed and when I next spoke to her, she told me that the sandalwood had cleared up most of the symptoms, leaving her with only an irritating discharge.

A visit to her local clinic, and subsequent tests, had shown that she had a trichomonas infection, and she was given antibiotics. The antibiotics prescribed cleared up the trichomonas but within a few days of finishing the course, my friend recognized the onset of thrush, which she described as 'a painless secretion of cottage cheese'. Not wishing to accept another course of antibiotics from the clinic, she once again came to seek my advice.

She is an intelligent woman, used to making her own decisions as to the way in which her body is treated, and when I told her that there were two oils which looked extremely likely to clear up the problem, she readily accepted, quite happy to be a human 'guinea pig'. **Niaouli**, reputed to be excellent for urinary infections, and which I had recently started using at home, was chosen, as I felt it would be powerful enough to take care of *candida*. Organically grown **lemon** oil, (which had cured a wart in just over a week) was mixed with the **niaouli**. I chose these two oils because Dr Valnet ascribes to them the properties which I felt were needed to combat thrush: **niaouli** is recommended internally for urinary infections, and **lemon** oil, Valnet says, 'activates the white corpuscles in the defence of the organism'. Also, intuitively, I felt that out of all the antiseptic, anti-fungal oils, these two would work well together.

I asked my friend to take three drops of each, in the morning and at night, knowing that it would either be helpful in clearing up the condition, or that it would have no effect, but that either way, it would cause no harm. Before taking the oils, the colour of her urine was a dark yellowish-orange and had an unpleasantly strong odour. Within days of taking the oils the urine became paler while, at the same time, the odour became less unpleasant. The oils were taken each day for two weeks at the end of which the thrush had gone completely, and the urine was a pale yellow colour with no unpleasant odour. Both my friend and I were overjoyed that the experiment had worked so well, and in such a short space of time.

Almost a year has passed since this treatment took place, my friend has not had a recurrence of thrush, and she feels that genitally she has a 'clean bill of health'.

I have spoken to many women who have suffered from thrush. Not only is it physically uncomfortable, but also emotionally disturbing. A woman may feel 'unclean' and her sex life is probably not enjoyable, or even nonexistent. This will put a strain upon a relationship if the situation continues for a long period of time. Clinical diagnosis of *candida albicans* is only the primary concern, since a woman with thrush is also likely to suffer from depression. It is interesting to note that researchers are now saying that depression is one of the contributing factors to a lowering of the immune system. It has also been proven that a weakened immune system is a contributing factor in the onset of *candida albicans.* We can see, then, that women are often caught in a vicious circle. In my opinion, essential oils can break that circle; first by fighting the fungal infection on a physical level, and then by lifting depression on an emotional level.

Note: **Sandalwood** oil has been shown in laboratory 'challenge tests' to be as powerful in its anti-bacterial action, as many of the broad spectrum antibiotics. Those French doctors who have also studied aromatherapy have perfected a system of testing which they call the 'aromatagram'. A culture is made from the patient's discharge and placed in petri dishes. One drop of essential oil (whichever essence is deemed to be the most appropriate) is added to each petri dish of culture and left for 24 hours. The effectiveness of the essential oil is measured by the size of the 'zone of inhibition'. This is the area of bacteria which has been killed by the essential oil within the time period.

Essences which have destroyed the largest areas of bacteria are then used to treat the patient. I find this method quite fascinating because there is no necessity to analyse and name the bacteria or fungus, but simply to find the essence or essences which will, quickly and effectively, kill the pathogen. (See 'Aromatherapy and the immune system' (page 76) for more details on *candida albicans.*)

PERIOD PAINS

Menstruation is not an ailment to be cured, as women are destined to bleed every month for a large part of their lives. However, the accompanying pain and discomfort can be alleviated with aromatherapy.

Sometimes the pain is only discernible on the first day of a period, and at other times it can drag on for several days, interfering with the enjoyment of everyday life. Occasionally the discomfort is so great that sufferers can only crawl off to bed and wait for a day or two until the worst of the pain has gone.

Over the years I have taken the recommended homoeopathic remedies, and although I experienced some relief from pain I still dreaded the 'monthly curse'. It was not until I became involved with aromatherapy that I truly could say 'I have found the solution to the monthly period pain.'

Clary sage oil was the essential oil which brought almost instant relief from pain and discomfort. There are two ways of using **clary sage** - internally or externally. My preferred method is to take two drops of **clary sage** oil in a teaspoon of honey with a little hot water - sipping the aromatic liquid at the beginning of the period when the pain is at its worst. Sometimes I would take a second dose a few hours later, but usually one dose was all that was required. For those who prefer to use essential oils only externally, **clary sage** can be used to cure menstrual pain by mixing a teaspoon of fatty oil with two drops of **clary sage** oil and massaging the lower abdomen, directly above the pubic hair-line. If aches and pains in the lower back are an accompaniment to the abdominal pain, then massage this area also. A third option is to make a hot compress (known as a fomentation) by adding a few drops of **clary sage** to a bowl of hot water (about 1 litre). Emerse a small towel in the liquid, wring it out, and apply to the lower abdomen. This obviously necessitates baring the skin and lying down for 15 minutes or so until pain relief is obtained.

Clary sage is a hormone regulator, which means that over a period of time the monthly periods may become completely painless, as mine did, so that pain relief is no longer needed. An added bonus is that **clary sage**, being a euphoric oil, lifts the heavy, depressed feeling which often accompanies 'the curse'.

As a teenager, I suffered badly from abdominal cramps and backache during every period, and only had recourse to codeine tablets and hot water bottles. If only I had known about **clary sage** when I was a teenager, I might have been more bearable to live with!

PREMENSTRUAL TENSION

Many women become tense and irritable a few days prior to the monthly 'curse'. Occasionally, women suffering with premenstrual tension have even committed murder, and because the concept of PMT is now medically accepted, some of these women were given lighter sentences due to 'diminished responsibility'. I experience a sort of insanity which can make me behave in completely irrational ways, and I can feel extremely vulnerable and cry at the slightest provocation. The oils of **clary sage**, **ylang-ylang** and **lavender** will be beneficial, whether used in the bath, or infused into the atmosphere of your room by placing a few drops on a source of heat. **Lemongrass** oil is strong and tangy, and I find that a **lemongrass** bath strengthens my emotions on those days when I am feeling emotionally wobbly. If bathing is not practical, I would put a few drops onto a tissue and carry it with me, keeping it within sniffing distance. **Rose** oil is calming and emotionally healing and this could be worn as a perfume for a few days, or it may be massaged into the solar plexus. **Rose** is excellent for soothing fraught emotions, and when used for controlling premenstrual tension, its uplifting aroma and powers of healing can bring immediate relief, making **Rose** a true 'woman's' remedy.

WATER RETENTION

Our body's ability to eliminate waste liquids is largely determined by the healthy functioning of our kidneys and lymphatic system. On those days of the month when water retention becomes apparent - when you can't get your jeans done up, or your skirt button has to be unfastened - a diuretic can be employed to help you feel comfortable again. Many foods (vegetables in particular) have diuretic properties and it is wise to eat healthily at this time. The essence which seems to work best as a diuretic is **juniper** oil, which may be used in the bath or a drop taken in honey water. Taken in small doses on the odd occasion (once a month) will not cause harm, but essential oils should not be ingested on a regular basis. Someone with chronic water retention has a systematic problem and should seek treatment from a qualified aromatherapist. A serious problem of fluid retention could indicate congestion of the lymphatic system.

CYSTITIS

This annoying and distressing problem is caused by an infection of the bladder or kidneys. Urinating is an unpleasant, often painful experience and the burning sensation when passing water is often accompanied by pain further up inside the abdomen. **Juniper** oil may be taken in honey water, or **sandalwood** oil rubbed into the kidney region of the lower back. If the discomfort is very bad, I recommend a sitz bath with **lavender** oil - after each visit to the toilet if this is practical. If you still have to go to work, then you could make up a bottle of **lavender** water to take with you (see page 141). A cotton wool pad soaked with **lavender** water applied after going to the toilet will give temporary relief and help you to maintain your sanity. All strong food and drinks should be avoided (tea, coffee, alcohol, spices), as should sugar and any foods containing sugar.

A friend of mine rang me in tears one Boxing Day, in agony with her cystitis. She had been treating it for some while, and had thought it was under control. However, Christmas temptations had lured her into drinking alcohol, and she was really suffering once again. Sex was out of the question, which was causing problems with her husband, and she was at her wit's end. I gave her a bottle of **juniper** oil with instructions to take one or two drops on a tiny amount of sugar, or in honey water, twice a day. After only two days she rang to say that it had worked miraculously, and everything was back to normal in her household.

VAGINAL DOUCHES

Candida albicans is the most common cause of vaginal irritation, and although *candida* is mentioned in more detail in another chapter, there are many people who prefer to douche rather than take essential oils orally.

Thrush is extremely irritating to the mucous membranes of the vagina, and can seem almost to drive you insane. In my early twenties I suffered recurrent bouts of thrush, and each time I visited my doctor I was given medicated pessaries which brought temporary relief only. I was never cured, and thought that perhaps I was destined to have thrush for the rest of my life. It was not until much later, after incorporating aromatherapy into my life, that I treated and cured myself of thrush. My choice of essences was **rose, lavender** and **bergamot** (see recipe chapter). I bought an enema pot from a chemist (or you may be able to buy a douche) and to 1 litre of warm water I added the essences, and douched twice a day. To ensure that the essences disperse, place them into a 100ml bottle of water and shake well. Transfer to the douche and top up with warm-hot water - a comfortable temperature for you. The relief from itching was apparent even from the first treatment, and I was pleased to know that the problem was diminishing. After a week of twice-daily douching, I reduced treatment to once a week for a further month. Douching should not be routinely employed as it will destroy the natural acid balance inside the vagina, but when used for periodic treatment of a particular complaint it is very beneficial.

HERPES

Herpes, being a virus, cannot be treated with antibiotics, and by and large it is thought to be permanent once it has caused infection through sexual intercourse. The virus is the same as that which produces cold sores. **Lavender, tea tree, lemon, sandalwood** and other essential oils which stimulate the immune system will aid your body to fight the virus. **Eucalyptus** sitz baths helped a friend of mine when the irritation became too great to bear. She was also given a **rose** blend to rub into the glands at the tops of her legs, and reported a marked improvement in her energy levels, together with a lessening of the pain. **Tea tree** oil could be applied directly to any blisters, as **tea tree** is very powerful in its action but will not irritate or harm the delicate skin of the vulva. As herpes tends to rear its ugly head when the body is under par - whether physically or emotionally - steps should be taken to enhance the immune system, thereby helping your body to keep the virus under control.

LEUCORRHOEA

A light vaginal discharge is quite normal, but prolonged, excessive discharge indicates that something is wrong. A tampon impregnated with **tea tree** oil may be inserted each night for a few days, or the discharge could be treated with a douche containing **lavender, bergamot** and **tea tree**. The vaginal discharge may be an indication of a food allergy, and suspect foods should be eliminated from the diet, at the rate of one per week. I have problems if I inadvertently eat dairy products while away from home, and as a preventive measure I regularly take two echinacea tablets each day. Echinacea is a herbal blood purifier.

PRURITIS

Pruritis means itching, and can pertain to the anus or the vagina. The saying 'there's no smoke without fire' could be translated as 'where there's an itch there's a problem'. An external irritant could be causing the irritation, and it is never advisable to spray perfumes or toilet waters near the vagina. Nor should you enter a bath to which essential oils have been added without first ensuring that they are thoroughly dispersed by agitating the water.

If the itching is very troublesome, a **lavender** sitz bath will bring relief. As with cystitis, washing the vulva after each visit to the toilet will soothe the skin and make you feel more comfortable. Sometimes the heat accompanying vaginal pruritis may cause the mucous membranes to be dry, thereby making sexual intercourse a little uncomfortable or painful. **Jojoba** oil makes a wonderful lubricant if sexual intercourse is uncomfortable due to the mucous membranes being dry.

CONDOMS

With increasing promotion towards safer sex the use of condoms is increasing. Many women find that the spermicidal covering causes irritation to the vagina. Although most condoms contain spermicide, there are some manufactured without, and if you experience this form of vaginal irritation it is advisable to use spermicide-free condoms. (Ask your pharmacist for advice.) Douching with **bergamot**, **lavender** or **tea tree** will help to remove traces of spermicide and help the vagina to return to normal. If preferred, a **tea tree** tampon may be inserted each night for two or three nights, until the vagina has healed. **Tea tree** is a powerful antiseptic, promoting the growth of new skin cells while being gentle on the skin; it is therefore the ideal oil to use for vaginal irritation. Condoms are disliked by many couples because they are too 'dry' and have an obviously 'rubbery' smell. Water-based lubricants are available in chemists, or use a little honey - one of nature's spermicides. Choose one which is delicately fragranced, if you are one of those people who finds the smell of rubber off-putting.

Chapter Three

SEXUALITY AND SENSUALITY

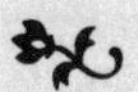

Healthy sexual organs are a prerequisite to full sexual expression. Who feels sexy when they've got thrush? Who wants to make love when they are experiencing the pain and discomfort of gonorrhoea? Genital health is important to our appreciation of sex and should be of primary concern. Because the genital organs have such sensitivity, we are equipped with a precision instrument by which we can monitor our body's health.

For example, if thrush did not cause itching and an unpleasant discharge, how would we know that we had a problem with *candida*? And if cystitis did not produce a burning pain on urinating how would we know that we had an infection of the bladder or kidneys? A painless discharge may well be overlooked, but it could indicate that we are allergic to a particular food, and we could reason that our body's reaction in this way is indicative of a problem on an internal level; a problem which we cannot see. We should be glad that our body is speaking to us, and then work towards finding and curing the cause of the problem, not just mitigating the symptoms; this is like ignoring the red warning light in your car, which is advising you that the oil level is dangerously low. You can either stop driving and buy a litre of engine oil, or you can continue driving and take the risk of wrecking the entire engine.

Clearing up any vaginal problems will certainly help you attain a relaxed and comfortable sex life. It is also important to be relaxed and comfortable with your method of contraception. If drugs and IUDs are abhorrent to you, the remaining choices are diaphragms and sheaths, not forgetting of course, rhythm, temperature charts, and abstinence.

Many more women would use sheaths and diaphragms if it were

not for the fact that the spermicidal covering can sometimes cause vaginal irritation and soreness. Of all the many and varied sheaths on the market, very few are free of spermicides, but there are some and your chemist will be able to give you advice. Sheaths are very often disliked by men, which then puts the responsibility for birth control with women. Many women use the diaphragm, which has other disadvantages, apart from needing to be used with spermicide; one that spontaneity is hampered as the diaphragm must be fitted in advance of intercourse, and removed after 8 hours. However, there is a new diaphragm which I have recently found out about, and which seems excellent. It is called the 'Honey Cap', and is one of the most 'natural' and unobtrusive methods of contraception. When not in use, it is placed in a pot of honey, and as honey is anti-bacterial this is the only form of protection it needs. The 'honey cap' is just rinsed in lukewarm water before insertion, and may be left in place for up to seven days at a stretch. During this time it is permissible to bathe and swim, which gives the wearer even greater freedom. The success rate of the 'honey cap' is comparable to the sheath or the regular diaphragm, but it would seem to me to offer women 100 per cent more freedom and confidence, and is absolutely perfect for those women (and their partners) who are sensitive to chemical spermicides or who wish to use a more 'natural' contraception.

APHRODISIACS

Assuming that our body is functioning properly, the next important factor is being 'in the right mood' and it is here that essential oils can play a useful and welcome role. Our sense of smell is closely linked to receptors in the brain which regulate the bodily functions, and of our five senses, it is the one which has the closest link to our emotions. We can be 'turned off' or 'turned on' by what we smell even more so than by what we see, after all it is easy to close our eyes and let imagination take over, but we cannot close off our sense of smell. Aromatherapy can literally 'spice up' your love life when certain essences are employed. There are many essences which excite the senses and register in the brain as being a 'turn on'; these include **ylang-ylang**, **jasmine**, **sandalwood**, **patchouli**, **rose** and **clary sage**. All of these essences make an ideal aromatic bath (aphro-matic bath) and may be used singly or in combinations of two or three. Just mix and blend until you find the aroma which is right for you. Sprinkling the essences around your room would be a beautiful way to 'create the right atmosphere', or add a few drops of your chosen oils to a bowl of hot water. Your favourite essence could also be worn as an all-over body perfume when added to **jojoba** oil, but an increasingly popular way to utilize the power of sensuous oils is by making your own massage oil. A massage between lovers is sensual and highly enjoyable, and when using a specially concocted massage oil (see recipe on page 143) to massage the back, legs, arms and so on, the result is physical relaxation and sexual stimulation. As the mucous membranes of the genitals are extremely sensitive, it is not advisable to use the massage oil in that area; however, the use of **sandalwood** here is completely safe, and will create a very pleasant sensation.

We are all sensual beings, created to give and receive pleasure, and each of us has an inbuilt flame of passion. Sometimes the pressures of surviving in this crazy world descend like a wet blanket to smother that flame, so that we can't imagine how good it was to be consumed by fire. When you are feeling this way, a long lingering **ylang-ylang** bath helps to remove that blanketed feeling, allowing you to feel once again, like a total woman.

Tea for Two!

I am not talking here about tea and biscuits with a neighbour while discussing the weather, but drinking an aphrodisiac tea when you are alone with your partner. Either green tea or black tea may be used, although green tea is preferable, owing to its delicate flavour and beautiful colour. One or two teaspoonfuls of tea leaves should be placed in a teapot. Put one drop of **jasmine** oil into the pot and add 3–4 cups of hot water. Serve immediately, and observe. The taste and aroma is exquisite and quite different from the jasmine tea which we can buy in packets from supermarkets. This is a practical and easily-made 'love-potion' and should be used with caution! A further caution must be to use only a quality essence. **Jasmine** is expensive to produce as well as to buy, and the obvious temptation to adulterate the oil must be considered. You probably will not be able to purchase good quality **jasmine** oil in the high street because of the high cost of the oil, but **jasmine** oil is available through reputable aromatherapy companies.

ANAPHRODISIAC

Just as certain essences can stimulate the senses, so the sedative oils can diminish them. I am sure that those people who do not believe in aphrodisiacs would also disbelieve the possibility of there being an anaphrodisiac. However, **marjoram** oil - as well as being a strong sedative - has the power to turn off sexual desire.

Marjoram may be diluted in a base oil for use in back massage; added to a bath for an evening soak; or a few drops sprinkled onto a burner so that the aroma is diffused into the room.

PERFUME YOUR LINGERIE

To give your lingerie your own 'personality', try adding one drop of your favourite essence to the final rinsing water, the next time you hand wash. Some oils, such as **patchouli** are a little too dark and heavy, but **ylang-ylang**, **geranium**, **myrtle**, **jasmine** or **neroli** will be fine.

You can scent your drawers and wardrobe with your favourite aromas. If you don't sew, simply sprinkle some essential oil onto a cotton-wool ball, place inside a greaseproof bag, prick holes in the bag and place it in a drawer, or pin it to the inside of your wardrobe. If you do sew, beautiful gifts could be made for friends or lovers, by making silk pomanders. Just cut a circle of silk or other light fabric (12 cm in diameter). Run a thread around the circumference, then place a ball of cotton wool sprinkled with your favourite essence or essences in the centre of the material, and gather the material, so that you have an aromatic ball. Finish off with a piece of narrow ribbon with which to suspend it from a clothes hanger. Use long-lasting scents such as **ylang-ylang, frankincense, sandalwood, patchouli, jasmine** or **rose**, rather than light citrus scents which are more volatile, and therefore less lasting. In Victorian times when cashmere shawls were imported from Kashmir in India, they were packed in boxes containing **patchouli** leaves, as the smell discouraged insects. The same is true today, and many essential oils will protect clothing from the ravages of moths.

Confidence Booster

A 'stiff drink' is the old standby for nervousness before going to a party, or meeting someone for the first time, but what does a non-drinker do?

You could take some Rescue Remedy, or else dab a little 'confidence booster' on the wrists or neck, or inhale the aroma from a bowl of warm water. For example, **jasmine** has the power to inspire strength and confidence in the wearer, and is one of the most exquisite and precious essential oils. In the time of the pharaohs of Ancient Egypt, only the privileged few would be able to wear such a fragrance, and even today **jasmine** is 'rare' in comparison to most other essences, which also makes it very expensive to purchase. However, a little goes a long long way, and because of the many special qualities it possesses, it makes a very good investment.

Breasts

Few women are truly happy about the size of their breasts, thinking that they are either too big or too small. The discontentment can cause feelings of insecurity and unhappiness, which can lead to an impairment of sexual pleasure. I am not saying that aromatherapy can automatically transform the breast size, but evidence has been put forward to suggest that some plants contain 'phyto-hormones' (plant hormones). These work in a similar way to human hormones, which are responsible for many functions, including the development of the breasts. **Geranium** oil is purported to be very rich in phyto-hormones and so, after a friend of mine had stopped breastfeeding her last child and found that her bust measurement had shrunk to 32 inches, I decided to put the theory to the test. **Ylang-ylang** was blended with **geranium** in a **sweet almond** oil base (see recipe on page 142) and given to her with instructions to rub it in night and morning, taking a few minutes to massage the muscles of the chest wall, directly above the breasts. An improvement in the size and tone of the breasts was noticed gradually, over a long period of time, but perseverence has paid off, because now her bust measurement is 36 inches, and the muscle tone is so good that a bra is an 'optional extra'.

Women who are well-endowed, but would prefer to be less so, could use **jojoba** oil with a little added **rose** oil regularly to gently massage the breasts. I have found that **jojoba** has the ability to emulsify fat deposits under the skin, which are then removed from the body. **Rose** is said to keep the breasts small and firm. **Jojoba** is an amazing liquid, having many unique properties which will be touched on in other sections of this book.

THIGHS

For many women the thighs are the area of the body they are least happy with. Diet alone will never remove unwanted fat from thighs, and exercise is very important, perhaps even more important than calorie counting. Certain essential oils, when massaged into the body, will aid the elimination of excess water and fat from thighs and buttocks. **Juniper** oil is a diuretic, which will tone up the circulation and help to detoxify the body. **Cypress** oil is an astringent, which when blended into a massage oil (see recipe on page 142), will firm and tone the muscles, which is desirable when one is losing weight, so that stretch marks do not become a problem. **Jojoba** oil will also help your body to remove superfluous fat deposits and toxins which have lodged in the tissues. The rate at which our metabolism works will largely determine whether or not we burn off the calories consumed, or whether those calories merely add to our size. Bodily sluggishness will result in a sluggish circulation and poor lymphatic drainage, in which case complete revitalization of the person will be necessary before slimming can hope to be successful. Being fat may cause some people to become depressed, and depression can slow down the rate of metabolism; so rather than reach for a 'comfort' cake or chocolate, make use of those essences that have uplifting qualities, and treat your emotions to the lift they deserve. Daily massage of the legs should always be in an upward movement (towards the heart), but keep it firm and gentle as the flesh should never be pummelled or pinched if cellulite is suspected - violent treatment will only make the condition worse. Cellulite is the 'orange peel' appearance of the skin, and is most often found on the thighs.

Making Your Own Perfume

Our sense of smell is the most direct way in which our emotions can be triggered. It is also, in many people, the most neglected of the five senses, and is often abused. Olfaction (to give it its technical term) is registered in our brain via the channels of the limbic system, and we react with pleasure or displeasure to aromas.

Once we have discovered that certain essences make us feel good and actually enhance our sense of well-being, it is rather nice to blend them into a perfume so that the subtle aroma can be with you every day, or just used on special occasions.

At one time, every perfume would have been skilfully blended from the finest essential oils, and would indeed have been a delight and an indulgence (on the psyche, and on the purse). Sadly, with the advent of laboratory created aromatic chemicals, perfumes have become more and more synthetic. Very expensive perfumes still use larger amounts of essential oils, having been created out of years of practice in the art of perfumery. Although unlikely to compete with these classic scents, you could make your own quite passable perfume using a few simple techniques of the perfumery trade (see page 143). You obviously will not be able to create a sophisticated perfume with long-lasting qualities, but you could enjoy making up your own 'signature'.

Essential oils are far too powerful to be worn undiluted, and a suitable base must be chosen. Alcohol is the usual medium in which a perfume is diluted, but pure alcohol is not for sale to the general public and alcohols such as vodka or gin, will make you smell like a cocktail. Vegetable oils, because of their oxidizing qualities are not suitable (because they go off), but **jojoba** oil, being a liquid wax, and not subject to oxidation, is the ideal base in which to dilute your mixture of essential oils. By keeping the blend very subtle, you could use it as an all-over body perfume, and because **jojoba** is so wonderful for the skin, you will have soft as well as delicately scented skin.

For hot summer days, you could have a lot of fun by making your own 'cologne'. A very simple blend of essences (see recipe on page 143) should be added to 'still' mineral water and shaken vigorously. During a heatwave, this delightfully refreshing cologne can be splashed on liberally, and should also serve to keep your mind alert and refreshed.

Create the Right Atmosphere

To create a light, euphoric atmosphere in preparation for a party, sprinkle **clary sage** around the room, or put a few drops into a bowl of warm water. Having lived and worked with essential oils for many years, I tend to take them for granted most of the time, but visitors always comment on the beautiful aromas and I certainly could not imagine my life without my essences. I would rather live with the scent of freshly picked flowers and herbs, than with the normal range of household smells.

Essential oils should be chosen according to the 'mood' of the party or the occasion. Here are some suggestions:

- **Bergamot**, **orange** and **rosewood** for a summer evening party

- **Frankincense, pine** and **orange** for a Christmas party
- **Ylang-ylang** and **rose** for a St Valentine's party
- **Sandalwood** and **patchouli** for a dinner party when the food is hot and spicy
- **Orange** and **lemon** for a children's party
- **Geranium** and **lavender** for an afternoon tea party
- **Rose** or **rosewood** for a teenage daughter's party.

The choice and the permutations are only subject to personal preferences and your budget.

TURN YOUR BEDROOM INTO A 'BOUDOIR'

With lashings of essential oils and a little imagination you can be Cleopatra, Madame Pompadour, or whoever you want to be. Essential oils and unguents were the only perfumes available in times gone by, because synthetic aromas had not been invented. The sails of ancient Egyptian barges were often drenched in aromatic oils and fragrant waters, and Cleopatra was reputed to have seduced Mark Anthony by wearing **jasmine** oil at their business meetings. **Rose** oil has always been highly prized and the Roman emperors were so fond of the aroma that they poured **rose** water into the canals running through their gardens.

Certain essential oils have 'heady', euphoric qualities, so why not take your favourites and imbue your bedroom with the magic and mystique of ancient civilizations. The heavier perfume notes of **rose, patchouli, jasmine** and **ylang-ylang** seem to be more suited to bedrooms and seduction, because their odour is on a level similar to that of natural body scent; the light citrus oils are reminiscent of the fresh outdoors and open spaces.

Rose must surely be the favourite perfume of all time. It has been used throughout the centuries, being mentioned in the *Kama Sutra* and *Perfumed Garden* and is still being incorporated into practically every high-class perfume. **Rose** otto has always been costly, and always will be so, due to the very small yield of essential oil from each flower; however, although the cost is high in comparison to that of other essential oils, it does 'keep' for a long time, and being so concentrated, a little could last for a very long time. **Rose** otto is distilled from the variety of rose known as *rosa damacena.* It is almost clear in colour and will solidify if placed in a refrigerator. Another **rose** which has many similar properties although solvent extracted from the variety of **rose** known as *rosa centifolia* (known as *rose absolute*). Both **rose** oils are regularly adulterated by profit-hungry companies, so be wary when seeking out a **rose** oil, and only buy from a reliable aromatherapy specialist. To my mind, **rose** is in a class of its own and no other scent makes me feel so special.

Chapter Four

MASSAGE

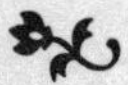

Cats loved to be stroked, dogs love to be patted, children to be cuddled - the sense of touch is important to all of us, but is not always fulfilled. Massage is one way in which the touch sensation can be enjoyed by another person, in a safe, unerotic way.

We are all sensual beings, in the same sense that a cat is sensual, and our bodies respond to and appreciate a massage. Whilst having a back massage, the recipient is being encouraged to let go of muscle tension, and thereby let go of stresses which may have built up in the muscles and tissues. Unless these tensions are released from muscles, the result is often pain, and then the remedy for controlling pain is often analgesic drugs such as paracetamol. It is unfortunate that the word massage has, over the years, become synonymous with prostitution and sleazy 'massage parlours'. However, a return to basic health matters, and a need to cope with the pressures of life today, has caused an upsurge in interest in massage as a therapy. The result is that now, for the first time this century, massage is becoming socially accepted as a legitimate 'hands on' therapy, alongside chiropractic and osteopathy. A massage with essential oils can be obtained from an aromatherapist, and even if you wish to massage your family and friends yourself, it is a good idea to experience a massage at the hands of a trained aromatherapist. In this way, you will feel how firmly to apply pressure, and how important warmth is to the recipient's overall enjoyment. The art of massage is essentially that of giving oneself to another person, and it is necessary to be healthy and full of energy before giving a massage. Sometimes one of my children might ask me for a massage, but if I am totally shattered from a hectic day, then I will postpone the massage until the following day.

The giving of a massage to someone you care for, whether partner, friend or child, is a beautiful experience, both for the giver and the receiver. It helps to have had a training in massage techniques, but this is not absolutely vital, as long as some basic rules are adhered to.

The recipient of the massage should be lying comfortably, and you should be positioned to the right or the left of the recipient, so that you are comfortable and can use your body weight to apply enough pressure without putting undue strain on your arms and back. The massage itself can take place just about anywhere that is comfortable, and ideally on a massage couch, but if this is not available, the next best place would be on a bed or on the floor; provided, of course, that you are not averse to kneeling for 30 minutes or so. I always use the floor on which to massage my children, having first made a makeshift massage pad with a padded beach mat covered by a large bath towel. A folded blanket would do just as well, making sure that it is the correct width and length for your 'patient'. Place a small pillow under the head and a regular sized pillow under the stomach of the recipient. A very plump person would probably not require the tummy pillow. Make sure that you have everything to hand that you will require: massage oil, tissues, and towels to keep the recipient warm, as you do not want to have to interrupt the massage to go away and fetch something.

There is a saying 'cold hands, warm heart', but when giving someone a massage, I can assure you that he or she will be more concerned about the temperature of your hands than of your heart. Cold hands will merely be interpreted as lack of consideration. So if you have cool hands prior to giving a massage, first immerse them in warm water for five minutes or so before beginning the massage. Rubbing your hands together will not make them feel warm to a hot back, although the friction brings some warmth to the palms of the hands. Never pour massage oil straight from the bottle on to someone's back, as it will shock the system. It is best to pour some oil into the palm of the hand, and then rub your hands together to disperse the oil evenly. Then place your hands on the

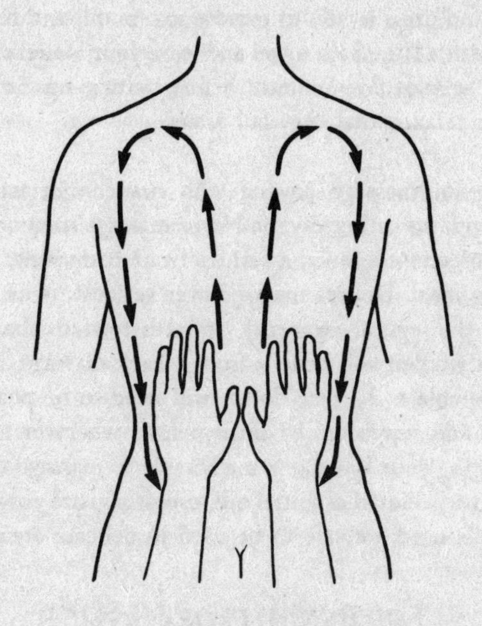

back of your 'patient' and distribute the oil evenly. With palms flat and fingers pointing towards the head of your 'patient' place your hands on their back at hip level, and slide them smoothly but firmly up the spine until your fingers reach the nape of the neck (See diagram). Draw your hands away from each other sideways across the shoulders, and glide your hands down towards the place from which you started. This movement, known as effleurage, should be carried out as one continuous movement, for at least 10 minutes. Next you should apply firm pressure with your thumbs and slowly work your way up the back to the shoulders, positioning your thumbs on either side of the spine, using the pads of the thumb and not the nail (see diagram above). Any sore spots located may be worked on for a few more minutes by rubbing the pad of the thumb in a circular motion across the sore area (never use the tips of the thumbs, otherwise your nails may cause discomfort to the 'patient'). Complete the massage with another 5-10 minutes of effleurage to soothe and relax. Cover the back with some kitchen towelling and press lightly to remove excess oil, and finally cover the back with a large bath towel and leave your 'patient' to remain prone for at least five minutes before getting up. Some people become so relaxed that they fall asleep.

Note: Do not massage anyone who has cancer, without first speaking with his or her doctor. Never massage someone who has an acute infection; a fever; a serious heart complaint; or has just eaten a big meal. Do not massage over varicose veins, and when massaging the legs, always work upwards towards the heart.

Pregnant women will benefit from a back massage, but as they will not be able to lie face down, will need to be positioned on their side, and supported by small pillows wherever necessary.

If massaging your lover, it is inadvisable to massage the genitals even with very diluted essential oils, unless you are absolutely sure that the oils used are safe to be used in delicate areas.

The Benefits of Massage

- Stimulates blood circulation, and circulation of lymph
- Stimulates the immune system
- Reduces tension
- Relieves muscle pain
- Is an acceptable way of giving TLC - tender loving care
- Soothes crying babies who have suffered a traumatic birth
- Enables diluted essential oils to be spread across a wide area of the body, and aids their penetration
- Helps children who are tense and can't sleep. Children are fed grown-up emotions - in TV programmes and on the news - with which they can't always cope.

TYPES OF MASSAGE

Full back massage - for general relaxation; to ease aches from over-exertion; to stimulate the immune system.

Hand massage for old people, when a back massage may not be appropriate. Many people automatically 'wring' their hands when under stress. Wringing of hands is therapeutic as there are as many reflexes on the hands as there are on the feet. To massage the hands of the elderly can bring comfort and release of tension.

Foot massage helps on many levels - it relieves aching, tired feet; gentle stimulation of the foot reflexes will generally be beneficial to the body; reduces heat and swelling of the feet, after prolonged periods of standing or walking.

Facial massage will relax your partner and help remove tension after a very stressful, upsetting day. Massaging the jaw line where much tension is stored (clenching of the teeth on an uncomfortable, crowded train; whilst sitting in a traffic jam; when the boss is being critical; etc) may prevent an outburst of negative emotion.

Massage of the upper back and shoulders - for insomniacs. A 10 to 15-minute massage before bedtime may help them to sleep without the need for tranquillizers. For a partner who wakes in the night, a five-minute massage may save you several hours of interrupted sleep.

Specialized areas. People who drive for long periods may require a massage of their upper arm; over-exertion during aerobics, dancing, etc, may require a leg massage, etc. People who sit at a desk all day may have a special need for a neck massage.

Note: When massaging the limbs, always work towards the heart.

CHECKLIST

- Remove your watch and any rings, as they may scratch the recipient and therefore detract from the general feeling of well-being.
- Make sure that your nails are not too long, especially the thumbnails. They should be short enough to allow you to massage with the pad of the thumb without the nail digging into the 'patient'.
- Have warm hands.
- Take the phone off the hook, if you don't have an answering machine.
- Dim the lighting - it is unpleasant to lie with a bright light shining in your eyes.
- Turn off the radio or television, so that the mind can also relax. Soft music in the background is sometimes beneficial if your 'patient' is uncomfortable in total silence.
- Make sure that you have everything you need before beginning the massage - massage oil; tissues; large towels - so that the continuity of the massage is not interrupted.
- Even in summer, ensure that the room is warm enough, as the body can cool down considerably during a 30-minute massage. You should wear something light and loose-fitting, such as a short-sleeved T-shirt.

Chapter Five

HEALTH AND HEALING

COLDS AND FLU

Many essences can be used to fight the common cold virus. Even **lavender** alone is good. My mother (who is now in her eighties) called me once a few years ago to say that she had a very bad cold and was worried that she might have to cancel her holiday (booked for one week's time). I told her to rub **lavender** oil under her jawbone, down the sides of the neck, on the muscles of the shoulders, and across the upper chest.

She rang again two days later to say that she was very much better, and that the pain in her shoulders (which was like a dull ache) had been eased as soon as the **lavender** was applied.

Here, it is safe to use the oil neat on the skin (unless of course, you have hypersensitive skin).

By using the essences in massage and in the bath, as is most popular in the UK and USA, we are helping our bodies to let go of stress and tension, both of which interfere with our appreciation of life. Too much stress will also lower our immune systems, making us more prone to illnesses.

I had not suffered from a cold for almost two years, until the week before I was due to fly around the world on business. The week before my intended departure, I developed a heavy cold, and as I had a meeting, which involved waiting for trains and taxis, by the time I arrived back home I was feeling pretty rotten. My symptoms were a very sore head, painful sinuses, and a very runny nose. My neck felt quite stiff, and my throat was sore. Determined not to 'get ill', and as I was too busy to take to my bed for a day, I set to work with my essences. **Lavender** was rubbed into my neck and to the base of my skull, and across the sinuses. **Sandalwood** was massaged under the jawbone (where there are lymph nodes), and internally I took three drops of **lemon** oil on a little brown sugar. At night I put a drop of **myrtle** oil on a tissue, and went to sleep with this across my nose and mouth, so that I was inhaling the vapours.

The next day I repeated the procedure, whilst working as normal, and when I awoke on the third day, my cold had gone.

Coping with Difficult Times

When we break a leg, we need a crutch to help us get around whilst the healing process takes place, and when the leg is once again strong and able to bear our weight, we throw away the crutch. It is the same when we are sad and troubled: we need a little something to help sometimes, to uplift us and make us feel better within ourselves, and about ourselves. So we can use **ylang-ylang**, or **rose**, or **clary sage** until we feel once again 'in control' of our emotions. Sadly, there are currently millions of people in the UK taking tranquillizers, most of whom needed a 'little bit of help' to see them through a particularly bad patch, but have since become addicted to the drug, and cannot manage without the tablets. This situation is rather like breaking the leg, using the crutch, but continuing to carry the crutch around for 5 to 10 years, so that it becomes a part of you. It is a crazy situation, and one which has to change.

Many people become so depressed that they go to their doctors for some advice. Nearly always the doctor will prescribe tranquillizers and sleeping tablets. Unfortunately, many of those people who had a case of acute depression are now addicted to the tranquillizers and cannot face life without them. So great is the problem that a recent survey revealed that 5 million people in the

UK are regularly taking tranquillizers, and many have been doing so for five years or longer. It is important that we can reach out for help when we need it, but just as when we break a leg we can use a crutch and then throw it away, it should be the same with depression. We can use essential oils to help us overcome our negative emotions, and then we can leave the essences in the bathroom. The large numbers of tranquillizer addicts makes me angry, because of the senseless prescribing of drugs which has lead to drug dependency - and what of the precedents we set for our children? (If mummy and daddy are 'hooked' on drugs, who can be surprised when little junior gets into drug taking?) We can only teach by our example.

I have definitely been in situations which have caused me mental anguish and depths of depression, but never have I consulted a doctor or desired to take tranquillizers. Always I have found help when I have reached for aromatherapy, whether I have gone to a friend for a massage, or made myself have an aromatic bath.

By tranquillizing our bodies, we are also tranquillizing our immune system, and are therefore less able to fight off the variety of illnesses which beset us. Whether those illnesses are caused by inhaling airborne bacteria and viruses, or whether we make ourselves ill by our own negative emotions, we are much more vulnerable when our immune system is not being allowed to work to full capacity.

And what of the prophylactic properties of essential oils? Aromatherapy is not just to treat an illness which has developed, but is also a protection from environmental pollution, as well as stress caused by our jobs, upsetting news stories, financial concerns, and insufficient sleep. Using essential oils in our day-to-day life is preventive medicine.

Stress

Executive burnout is on the increase in many countries, and although a certain level of stress is beneficial and leads to better results, too much leads to executive burnout with resultant ill-health. If the daily stress is attended to in the same way as the daily hygiene is attended to, then we do not allow a buildup of stress to put an unacceptable load on our body and mind.

Anyone who owns a car will be aware of the need to check the engine oil at regular intervals, and to have the car serviced regularly. Are humans less important than cars? All too often in this materialistic world, we find ourselves working for companies that have structured their working methods for economic costs and economic benefits. We should be looking at human costs and human benefits.

Of course we have our obligations to fulfll, but we also have an obligation to ourselves. We are not machines, and we need to take care of our bodies not just so that we can function efficiently, but so that we can appreciate the wonder of life, and the source of life.

Stress is a very big problem in the world, where we have duties and obligations. The stress in our bodies can build up to such an extent that we suffer 'dis-ease'. The human body cries 'enough', and then all of our responsibilities and duties have to be taken care of by someone else. I have a lot of stress in my life, what with running my own business, writing books, and travelling around the world giving lectures, as well as caring for three children. The secret of staying on top of it is to unwind in a deep, hot bath, to which I have added some of my favourite essences, and to incorporate essential oils into my home life as much as possible. Breathing in the aromas of nature makes me feel beautiful and tranquil, and I forget the cares of the day. To me, the essences are one of God's gifts to us, and by inhaling their beauty into us, they help us to experience the beauty of life once again. I also tend to live my life with a Scarlett O'Hara philosophy of 'tomorrow is another day', finding that if I try to take on too many worries at once, then I don't manage to cope very well with any of them. What always amazes me is that no matter what traumas I am going through, or how mentally fraught I feel, people invariably tell me that I am looking good.

WARTS AND VERRUCAS

My experience of curing warts and verrucas is with children and you will find details of which essences to use in the chapter on 'Childhood illnesses' (Chapter 10).

ATHLETE'S FOOT

Food allergies often play havoc with the immune system, and I have mentioned elsewhere that my son has an allergy to dairy products. It was easy to keep him away from milk products when he was young, and I had hoped that he would never be tempted to try any, but at the age of 14 he started eating ice creams and chocolate bars whilst out with his schoolfriends. I was unaware of a problem until the day he complained of a sore foot and showed me the problem. The ball of his foot and his toes were swollen and there were areas of dead skin between his toes - there was no doubt that it was athlete's foot. It was quite advanced before I ever saw it, and was well into the dermis (second layer of skin). For two days I used **lavender** footbaths, and put **tea tree**-impregnated lint between the toes. James has very sensitive skin, and is one of those people who is sensitive to **tea tree**. As the **lavender** was not clearing the athlete's foot, and I was becoming more concerned at the spread of the fungal infection, I took my son to our doctor, who prescribed a hydro-cortisone cream. It was applied that night, but by the next morning the foot was puffed up like a balloon, and I decided that with an adverse reaction like that, and as my essences were not working, I had better contact my ex-husband.

A weak **garlic** oil solution was made in a base of **sweet almond** oil. Actually, when speaking of garlic, there is no such thing as 'weak' and even at 0.5 per cent strength, the entire house reeked for a long time. Within two days, the spread of the fungus had been arrested, and healing had begun. Dressing the foot had to be done every 3-4 hours, as the heat and itching became intolerable, sometimes preventing James from sleeping at night. A **lavender** footbath was used first, for about 5-10 minutes, and the old lint carefully removed. Neat **lavender** oil was used to sterilize the scissors and tweezers with which I trimmed away the dead skin. Then after gently drying the foot, **garlic**-soaked lint was placed between and around each infected toe and secured with micropore tape and the entire foot was encased in an envelope of cotton material. Day by day the infected area grew smaller, with new skin growing in its place, and after a while, I noticed that the **garlic** was causing the new skin to blister and peel. This is when I stopped using the **garlic**, and reverted to using **lavender**-impregnated lint between the toes. It took several weeks to bring James back to a state of health, during which time he was given high doses of vitamin C, echinacea tablets, and herbal teas, and he was not allowed to eat any foods containing yeast.

Garlic, as a powerful healer, has been known about for a very long time, either when taken internally or used externally. A friend of mine related the story to me of how someone he knew cured athlete's foot by crushing up a lot of **garlic**, putting it into a plastic bag, and then putting his foot into the bag and leaving it on overnight.

CHEST INFECTION

The following is an extreme case of how essential oils have the strength and the power to fight a serious infection, even when conventional medicine had failed to work. The case history is particularly impressive because the person with the infection was in a coma, and therefore there was absolutely no possibility of any other influence such as 'positive thinking' or 'mind over matter' being responsible for the cure. This story was related to me by an acupuncturist friend of mine, who was the 'therapist' in this case. (Prior to studying acupuncture she was a State Registered Nurse.)

A friend of my friend was involved in a bad car crash, which resulted in a protracted hospital stay on a ventilator. The crash victim was in a coma for several weeks and was being kept alive by machinery. A chest infection worsened to such an extent that the hospital doctors tried every drug possible to clear up the respiratory problems, but still there was no response. The parents were informed that their daughter would probably not pull through, and it was at this time that my friend asked the permission of the parents and the hospital consultants to use some alternative remedies. Because of the ventilator, my friend was not able to use her acupuncture needles, but she rubbed some **tea tree** oil into the chest area, and also added drops of **tea tree** to the receptacle on the ventilator. **Tea tree** was administered in this way for several days, after which period of 'intensive care', the chest drained of fluid (a dark brown colour). From then on the patient's health improved tremendously; she came out of the coma, and is now back at home with her parents and on the road to making a full recovery.

Tooth Abscess

In the spring of 1989 I developed what I thought was toothache, and thought I had better see my dentist. I soon discovered that I had in fact got an abscess at the base of my eye tooth. It became swollen and painful, as well as hot. The normal treatment for a tooth abscess is antibiotics, but not wishing to take antibiotics, I applied **clove** oil because I knew it to be efficient for the treatment of toothache, and that it is also slightly anaesthetic. I was not sure whether the **clove** oil might in fact be a little too strong for the skin in my mouth to tolerate, but found that there was no adverse reaction. The **clove** lessened the discomfort, producing a warm, slightly numbed feeling. I continued to apply the **clove** oil, 2-3 times a day, for almost three weeks, until the abscess had shrunk and my gum was again normal. All that was left to remind me was a tiny 'raised spot' on my gum. I realize that antibiotics would probably have worked much faster than the **clove** oil, but I have the patience to wait for three weeks for a cure, and the satisfaction of being shown again how powerful the essential oils are. I also have the satisfaction of knowing that yet again I have been able to avoid a course of antibiotics, and therefore have not compromised my immune system.

Note: **Clove** oil is a skin irritant and should not be allowed to come into contact with the lips or the facial skin. Should this happen accidentally, apply a liberal coating of vegetable oil in order to dilute the essential oil.

Tranquillizers - How to Come Off Them

A woman in her thirties was introduced to me a few years ago. She was a heavy smoker and had been taking Ativan tablets three times a day since the birth of premature twins. One had died, and the other had survived with the aid of a ventilator. She realized that her heavy smoking had been a contributing factor in the death of her child, and this knowledge created terrible guilt feelings, leading to depression. It was because of the depression that the Ativan tablets had been prescribed, but after three and a half years, she had come to terms with the situation and wanted to 'come off' the drugs.

I suggested that she cut out the night-time tablet - instead substituting a **lavender** bath, and also add a drop of **lavender** to the edge of the pillow if she felt the need. She did this for two weeks, and feeling good, and pleased with herself, she wanted to cut down on the other tablets. I gave her **clary sage** and **ylang-ylang** to help her confidence and combat her depression, and these were to be used during the day, either in the bath or in a bowl of hot water to scent the atmosphere. I also made up a diluted **jasmine** in **jojoba** blend to wear as a perfume, for those days when things 'started to get on top of her'.

Within two months of wanting to come off Ativan, she had succeeded - with a little help from aromatherapy. She was feeling so good at having quit Ativan that she decided to stop smoking, as she wanted to have another baby. With her own self-determination plus the help of aromatherapy, over a period of a few months she managed to stop smoking, and one year later she gave birth to a healthy baby.

Slimming

Essential oils can act as wonderful slimming aids to the serious slimmer, provided that diet and exercise are also attended to. A sluggish circulation and water retention are problems which are often taken for granted by an overweight person, as is a slow metabolism. **Juniper** oil is a natural diuretic, and will help the body to excrete excess water. **Juniper** may be taken internally, in small amounts (one or two drops on sugar each day) for a short period of time, which will cause an increase in the flow of water from the body. Along with the liquid goes toxic waste that, unless eliminated, builds up in the tissues of the seriously overweight person. Alternatively, **juniper** may be used in combination with **cypress** in a massage oil, or in the bath. The diuretic properties of **juniper** and the astringent properties of **cypress** create a perfect 'slimming oil' (See recipe on page 146.) Women with small breasts but large hips should take a **juniper** hip bath. Just sit in a bath to which you have added six inches of water, and six drops of **juniper** oil, but do not lie down as you don't want to lose any weight from the breasts.

Fat people tend to get depressed about their weight and, feeling that they can do nothing about it, seek comfort in eating foods which they know will not improve their shape and size. It is a vicious circle which can be broken by not giving in to temptation, but when an eating binge threatens, take a **clary sage** and **ylang-ylang** bath instead. The uplifting aromatic waters may just give you enough of a lift to make you proud of yourself, and confident that you have it in your own power to change the way you look.

Regular bathing with essential oils will improve the tone of the entire body, and the clarity of the skin, and can increase the metabolic rate and generally make you feel fitter and more determined to 'fight the flab'.

Take Your Healthy Atmosphere with You

Hotel rooms seem to me to be the ideal place to catch a variety of diseases, depending on what was wrong with the previous occupant. Whenever I need to stay in a hotel, I always take with me a selection of essential oils, and never feel 'safe' until I have sprinkled them around the room and in the bed. My personal preferences are **rosewood, bergamot** and **lavender**, but if the weather is cold and damp and the room is chilly, then I sprinkle **myrtle** oil around the room, as I find the aroma to be warming and strengthening. **Bergamot** oil, being green in colour, will stain white surfaces, so I am always discreet with my use of essential oils. As a non-smoker, I like to make use of hotel ashtrays by filling them with hot water and adding a few drops of an essential oil, but I may not be able to do this for much longer as more hotels offer non-smoking rooms.

Other essential oils which would help to purify the atmosphere would be **tea tree**, **niaouli**, **lemon**, **eucalyptus**, and **rose**, and if you just want to feel 'home from home' then take along any of your favourite essential oils.

Mouth Ulcers

Mouth ulcers generally occur when one is run down or when there has been an excessive consumption of sugar-laden foods. Christmas is a common time to find that you have a mouth ulcer, due to over-indulgence in rich, sugary foods. It is easy to tell if you have a mouth ulcer as soon as anything sweet goes into your mouth, as the ulcer will begin to hurt. So the first thing is to eliminate sweet foods from the diet until the ulcer has healed. **Myrrh** or **tea tree** oil are two very good oils for curing mouth ulcers. I like to use **myrrh** oil, and apply it to the ulcer on the tip of a cotton bud. However, many people find the taste and smell of **myrrh** quite repulsive, and therefore **tea tree** oil will be suitable for them. If neither of these oils is available or they are disliked, then **lavender** oil will work very well also. Whichever essence is chosen, a slight stinging sensation will be experienced on first applying it to the ulcer, but the discomfort will quickly turn to relief. When essential oils are used two or three times a day, the mouth ulcer will normally disappear within a day or two.

SPOTS

We are all occasional victims of the facial spot. It seems to erupt just before we have to go somewhere special, or look our very best. Sometimes spots occur just before or at the start of menstruation, when there are hormonal changes happening within the body. Clogged pores are often responsible for facial spots, and this can be prevented by daily attention to thorough skin cleansing. (See page 91 about acne.) Food allergy is another classic reason for facial spots, and eating problem foods should be avoided. I know that I am allergic to dairy products, and so eliminate them from my diet. However, I occasionally take a decision to eat some forbidden food, whilst away from home. This could be an innocent-looking pat of butter at breakfast in a hotel, or a portion of dairy ice cream, or on those occasions when I feel like having a dessert and there is nothing available without cream. When I have eaten some forbidden food I automatically take extra quantities of echinacea tablets, as these blood purifiers help my body to eliminate the allergen, but sometimes a spot still manages to break through. Then I take a cotton bud dipped in **lemon, tea tree, niaouli, lavender** or **eucalyptus** - whatever I have handy - and apply directly to the spot. This first-aid treatment often banishes spots overnight, but definitely within a few days the spot will have gone. Also at this time it is important to drink large quantities of pure water, to help the cleansing process, and of course, to monitor the diet carefully, so that further allergens are not taken into the body.

SUNBURN

The majority of us, at some time or other, have probably been unlucky enough to suffer the agonies of sunburn, and whilst slapping on the après-sun lotions, have vowed never again to underestimate the burning rays of the sun. I learnt my lesson at the age of 19, after falling asleep on a beach in Ibiza. My back was so red, and the skin so delicate, that just to touch it resulted in broken skin and absolute agony. I remained in a hotel room feeling sorry for myself for the remainder of my holiday, not knowing then about the wonders of aromatherapy. I only wish I had been given some **lavender** or **tea tree** oil all those years ago, and nowadays I carry a bottle of **lavender** oil at all times. **Lavender** and **tea tree** both have amazing properties to soothe and heal burned skin. These two essences may be used neat on small areas of sunburn, but for a large area such as a burnt back, the essences should be diluted first. A fatty oil is inappropriate here, as fatty oils will hold in the heat, and make you feel even worse. Therefore, the **lavender** or **tea tree** should be diluted in water, and can be used in concentrations far stronger than those for facial skin cleansers or tummy compresses. To a litre of water, add 5ml of **lavender** or **tea tree**, and shake vigorously. Smooth material, such as a cotton handkerchief (a towel will feel far too 'prickly' for comfort), should be saturated with the lotion and applied to the burn, and this treatment repeated as soon as the cloth becomes dry. This treatment will take out a lot of the heat, and soothe the burnt skin, and on reaching home or hotel, a tepid bath to which a few drops of **lavender** or **peppermint** have been added will be beneficial. An alternative to the compresses could be to fill a plant mist spray with lukewarm water plus a few drops of **lavender** oil, and spray over the sunburned areas. It will bring immediate relief and can be repeated as often as required. At this time, alcohol should be avoided as your body desperately needs water to repair the damaged skin tissue, and alcohol will rob the body of fluids. So drink plenty of water and save the alcohol for a celebration when your burn has healed.

Note: With the exception of applying neat essences to spots, the only essential oils which should be used neat on the skin are **lavender** and **tea tree**. (A few people are intolerant of **tea tree**, and therefore they should only use **lavender** for the treatment of burns.)

SKIN PIGMENTATION

A few years ago, my youngest daughter returned from a two-week Spanish holiday with her father and the sight of her skin really upset me. On her normally tanned face she had large white blotches and on her upper chest, arms and back there was a combination of raw red skin, blisters and dead wrinkled skin. Where the skin had blistered and the blisters joined together, the skin had peeled off leaving areas of pigmentation more than two inches in diameter. My daughter was feeling really miserable, not only because she was in pain but because she was disfigured (although only on the surface layers of the skin) and she was afraid it would be permanent. Whether the skin's reaction was an allergy to the sun itself or to a suncream I will never know, but as it is not possible to go back in time and alter events I just set about the process of making my daughter feel better. Whilst she was soaking in a lukewarm **lavender** bath I mixed up a blend of fatty and essential oils - blending together the ingredients which I felt would be most beneficial. For the base I chose **camellia** oil as it is quickly absorbed by the skin and does not leave a greasy feel, very important when it was going to be applied several times a day. Combined with the **camellia** oil was a little **rosehip** seed oil as it has a reputation for being a skin rejuvenator, and having used it in my own skincare routine I knew that it was indeed a fast-acting skin regenerator.

The essential oils chosen were **lavender, niaouli, rose, tea tree** and **sandalwood. Lavender** because it is the best remedy for sunburn as well as being gentle and soothing to inflamed and irritated skin. It also promotes the growth of new skin. **Tea tree** was added as it is renowned as a healing agent in the case of a burn and has an inhibitory action on germs. **Sandalwood** has been used for centuries to treat dry skin and helps the skin to retain moisture - a very important consideration after sunburn. **Niaouli** oil, as well as helping to heal burns, is antiseptic and as some of the broken blisters were becoming infected I needed something which was gentle on the skin but yet powerful enough to cope with the threat of sepsis in a large expanse of raw skin. **Rose** was chosen in part for its soothing, healing and antiseptic properties but also because its aroma is so uplifting and inspiring, and I knew that it would help to banish the look of misery etched into my daughter's face and make her feel better in herself and more confident that the pain and disfigurement were only temporary. Whilst I was mixing up the special blend, my daughter relaxed in her lukewarm **lavender** bath, and after very gentle drying off the aromatherapy blend was applied. Every day, in conjunction with taking an evening **lavender** bath, the oil mixture was applied several times. Within two weeks of commencing treatment there was a 50 per cent improvement.

My daughter was dreading the first day of school in September even though the acute 'burn and blister' stage had passed and she was feeling very much better, because she thought she would be teased by her classmates. Although she did get rather bored with having to explain her mottled appearance, she handled the situation very well. I continued to apply the special blend to her skin (gradually reducing the frequency of application down to once a day) and by the time her school broke up for the half-term holiday, her skin had healed, the pigmentation was no longer visible and the horrors of the summer holiday were no more than a distant memory.

FOOTBATHS

Relief from hot aching feet can be obtained by adding a few drops of **peppermint** oil to a bowl of lukewarm water (or sit on the edge of the bath with a few inches of water in the bottom) and let the feet soak for 15 minutes. **Peppermint** is very fast acting because it contains natural menthol, which is incredibly cooling (Also see pages 21-22.)

HEADACHE

Headaches are such a common occurrence in the Western world that they have become big business for the drug companies, who are always claiming a new fast-acting remedy, and will spend millions of pounds in promoting it on television. Often, headaches are caused by neck tension, which is hardly surprising when you consider the weight of our heads which have to be supported by the neck, and it is the muscles at the back of the neck which are put under incredible strain every time we sit at a desk and pore over books, whether at school, college, or office. Headaches resulting from overstrained neck muscles can be alleviated quickly and safely by rubbing a little **lavender** oil into the muscles of the neck. This makes much more sense than swallowing aspirins or paracetamol drugs, which have first of all to be digested, and then assimilated into the bloodstream, and then to travel to the brain where the pain is registered, and dull the pain. Another common cause of headache is eyestrain, and again **lavender** will help when it is gently rubbed over the temples and forehead. Sometimes though, the cause of the headache must be recognized, and avoiding steps taken. There are two ways in which I get headaches. One is if I am driving a long distance, and push myself to drive too far in one day, with the result that I do not eat properly and do not take sufficient rest. A headache then tells me that I simply have to take a break. Similarly, when I am working at my computer for long periods of time, I know in theory that I should take a five-minute break every hour. I rarely do this, until my head begins to throb like an internal alarm clock: 'time to get up, and walk away from this machine'. Then I go out for a walk in the fresh air, or put a few drops of some relaxing essence onto my burner, and lie down for 20 minutes.

When a headache is accompanied by nausea, then whether or not it is labelled as a migraine the best remedy is a dose of **peppermint** oil in honey water. When this mixture is sipped from a spoon, the relief from both the nausea and the headache is rapid. Even **peppermint** oil on a tissue, sniffed frequently, will dispel a headache caused by overeating or indigestion. Sometimes though, the best cure for a headache is just to give up and go to bed for a good sleep, aided by a drop or two of **lavender** oil on the edge of the pillow.

INDIGESTION

Indigestion can have a variety of causes - a hastily eaten meal, eating on-the-trot through lack of time, or eating a meal late in the evening and then going to bed before the food has been digested. For very fast relief from the discomfort of indigestion, take one drop of **peppermint** oil on a sugar lump, or preferably in honey water (one teaspoon of honey and two-three teaspoons of hot water). I find that warm honey water enables the **peppermint** oil to work very quickly, as the essence reaches the bloodstream faster. There are very few guarantees in life but peppermint has, so far, never failed to work for me when I have been unable to sleep or have felt sick due to indigestion. Flatulence can also be treated with oil of **peppermint** taken on sugar or in honey water. One drop of oil to a small glass of water into which half a teaspoon of honey has been stirred, will usually do the trick. However, flatulence often accompanies constipation; anyone suffering from constipation should massage their buttocks.

TOOTHACHE

The age-old remedy of **clove** oil being used for toothache holds just as good today as it did decades ago, and although most essential oils have been dropped from the British Pharmacopoeia, **clove** oil continues to be listed, and sold by most chemists. **Clove** has a slightly analgesic effect, and numbs the nerves in the local area of application. A drop on cotton wool or a cotton bud should be applied to the affected tooth every day until either the pain goes away or you can visit a dentist for treatment. **Peppermint** oil is also a good remedy for toothache when applied to the affected tooth.

HAEMORRHOIDS (PILES)

Haemorrhoids are very painful and although many people have had piles or currently are suffering, everyone suffers in silence, hoping that the piles will go away, and too embarrassed to talk about the problem. Surgical removal is an all-too-common means of removing the problem, but this drastic method should only be accepted as a last resort. **Cypress** oil is a natural astringent, and will shrink piles almost as if by magic. Friends have told me that their piles have simply shrunk and disappeared after a **cypress** bath (five drops of **cypress** to a bowl of warm water). A sitz bath should be taken once a day until the piles have gone. Please do not be tempted to apply **cypress** oil neat, as it is very strong and will only cause further discomfort. It is sensible to take a litre bottle of water, to which you add 20 drops of **cypress**, shake the mixture well, and use some of the mixture every time you take a sitz bath. Shaking the drops in a bottle of water ensures that they are well dispersed. Haemorrhoids often occur if the person is constipated, and so pay attention to your diet. All sugary foods and bleached flour products should be replaced with wholemeal products and fresh vegetables. Sufferers from haemorrhoids could take a small bottle of the **cypress** mixture or **lavender** water to work with them and apply it on a cotton wool pad in the rest room.

HIGH BLOOD PRESSURE (hypertension)

As **lavender** oil is sedative and has been attributed with the ability to lower blood pressure, I have recommended it to several people suffering from high blood pressure. My mother, who suffers from hypertension, takes regular **lavender** baths, and has, for a long time, not needed to take the doctor-prescribed drugs for this condition. Of course, it is not always convenient for my mother to take a **lavender** bath, and whenever something has occurred to upset her or make her feel 'hot and bothered', she puts a little **lavender** oil on a tissue and inhales the vapours for a few minutes. Of course, you should not stop taking your prescribed drugs without first consulting your doctor. Because of **lavender**'s powerful action in lowering blood pressure, it should *not* be used by people known to be suffering from hypo-tension (low blood pressure).

INFLUENZA

I find that influenza responds very quickly to homoeopathic remedies but when these are not readily available, there is an aromatic treatment which has the ability to abort a cold and shorten an influenza attack.

Fill a bath with comfortably hot water. Mix a quantity of **lavender** oil in a base oil (see page 147), and rub the mixture into your body, paying particular attention to the chest area and back of the neck, then jump into the bath and soak for about 10 minutes or so. Dry quickly, and go straight to bed. This treatment will usually lessen the severity of the attack, and in some cases it clears up the symptoms overnight. The **lavender** is being pushed into the body by the heat of the bathwater, where it will begin to kill the invading organisms, and at the same time to boost the immune system to produce more antibodies and white blood cells. Several other essential oils will fight a cold virus, and these are **sandalwood**, **myrtle**, **niaouli**, **tea tree** and **lemon**. Either singly *or* in combination, these essences should be employed in a night-time bath.

RELIEF FROM SEVERE FLU SYMPTOMS

It's a Knockout was once the title of a television programme but today it could easily be the name given to the current strain of influenza. I have had flu many times during my lifetime, but the latest flu 'bug' really did knock me off my feet. Exactly one week before the launch of my new book I woke up in pain and discomfort and realized that I had not been having a nightmare in which I was being tortured, but the pain in my head and agonizingly stiff neck were symptoms of 'the flu'. Not being able to move my head around the pillow without experiencing almost unbearable pain, I decided that if a hangover was anything like this then I would certainly never want to drink alcohol again. I had a 10am appointment, which I valiantly kept, but then decided to give up on everything and go to bed. Over the next 36 hours I slept, drank bottled water and rubbed essential oils into various parts of my body.

Lavender, that good old standby, was rubbed into the nape of the neck and top of the head, in order to bring some relief from the headache and stiff neck - which it did. Usually with flu there is a lethargy accompanied by pains in the spine and extremities, but on this occasion there was a difference. The calves of my legs were so painful that if I had run a marathon race it is doubtful whether they could have felt any worse. Similarly, my upper arms felt as though I had been weight-training for several hours at a stretch and the muscles were sore to the touch. But overriding the pain and discomfort was the feeling of complete and utter exhaustion and I could not help thinking 'this must be what it feels like to be dying'.

I lay in bed thinking about my essential oil collection and wondering which essence would be best for my condition. Influenza is caused by a virus, that is common knowledge, and it is also common knowledge that viruses have to be killed by the body's own defence systems. Knowing, however, that certain essential oils can aid the body's fight, and feeling that the pain in my calves and arms was due to the presence of a virus, I decided to apply diluted **ravansara** oil. **Ravansara** is botanically related to bay laurel, and smells vaguely similar. It grows in Madagascar and Australia and is one of the oils employed by French doctors in their aromatic treatment of viral infections, especially of the respiratory tract. I added 2ml of **ravansara** to a 100ml bottle of **camellia** oil, and liberally rubbed the problem areas - legs, arms and neck.

By the following morning I was feeling sufficiently well to carry out my normal daily tasks, and I was relieved to think that I would be able to cope with the week ahead, which consisted of one newspaper and three radio interviews plus a book-signing session. During the day I was speaking to a teacher of aromatherapy when I happened to mention that I was just getting over flu. She asked me if I had used **tea tree** oil on the soles of my feet, and recommended that it be used neat. Essential oils are so versatile that there is always more to learn and understand and I am always open to trying something new. For the next few days I could be seen periodically removing my socks in order to anoint the soles of my feet with neat **tea tree** oil. Once again, aromatherapy came to my rescue and with the prudent use of **lavender, ravansara** and **tea tree** I was able to resume working within days of falling ill. I have to admit, though, that my brainpower took considerably longer to return to normal - 'the lights are on but there's nobody home' definitely applied to me that week, but nevertheless I was at least able to keep to my book-launch schedule.

GASTRIC FLU

A few days after reading newspaper reports that the Queen and other members of the Royal Family had been struck down with gastric flu, I too became a victim of one of the many epidemics to have swept the UK in the early 1990s.

I had gone to bed feeling fine, only to awaken in the early hours of the morning with a violent headache and intense nausea. The **lavender** oil which I rubbed into my head and neck greatly reduced the headache but did little to allay the nausea or the vomiting of bile. Half-heartedly I thumbed through my *Materia Medicia* looking for a homoeopathic remedy, but my headache got the better of me and I soon gave up the task and staggered to the kitchen where I made myself some **peppermint** and honey water. To a teaspoon of honey I added two drops of **peppermint** oil, stirred it well and then added half a cup of hot water, which I took back to my bed and sipped intermittently. **Peppermint** oil is very comforting to the stomach, soothing the nauseated feeling whilst taking away the nasty taste which is invariably left in the mouth. It also helps to reduce the fever which often accompanies a gastric upset. Every time I turn to **peppermint** oil when feeling sick or suffering from acute indigestion, I am always amazed and grateful at the speed of recovery.

Peppermint has been known as a stomachic for hundreds of years, when it was generally prescribed as a 'tea'. Although **peppermint** in large amounts can be an irritant to the intestinal tract, in small amounts we come into contact with it every day of our lives. Almost all toothpastes contain **peppermint** oil and it is a common ingredient in many mouthwashes. It is also commonly used in confectionery and is the familiar flavouring in chewing gums and 'mints' - with or without a hole.

A pure **peppermint** is a 'must' on my kitchen shelf and is one of the essences which I would want with me if ever marooned on a desert island. But care must be taken when purchasing **peppermint** oil to ensure that it is pure - the best variety is *mentha piperata*. There are many varieties of mints available such as *mentha spicata* and *mentha arvensis* (which is the major flavouring agent of toothpastes), but these are inferior in terms of fragrance, flavour and potency.

SEE THE GOOD WITHIN THE BAD

Nobody ever wants to get flu or spend a whole day vomiting - I certainly don't ever consciously wish to get sick - but often an acute illness is a blessing in disguise. For example, when writing my last book and working long into the night, I got into a bad habit of drinking coffee, and although I tried very hard to 'give up', the best I could manage was to reduce the number of cups I drank down to one cup per day. No matter how I tried I just could not let a morning slip by without brewing myself a fresh pot of coffee. Then the 'flu bug struck, and a cup of coffee was the very last thing I desired. I naturally increased my intake of mineral water as I found that I felt thirsty all of the time, and even since recovering I have continued to drink lots of mineral water and have lost my 'need' for coffee. I recently drank a cup of coffee to see if I would still enjoy the taste, but found that I no longer even enjoyed the aroma. We are such creatures of habit - which is good news for the coffee companies but not good news for us - because breaking with that habit can be difficult. What better time, then, to throw off those ingrained habits - smoking, drinking coffee, over-indulgence in alcohol - than at the same time when our body is throwing off an illness? I am becoming more aware that illness and health are just like 'yin' and 'yang' and that there is always bad within the good and good within the bad. If we can see today's illness in a positive way, it will give us more control over tomorrow's health.

LARYNGITIS/SORE THROAT

Any inflammation of the throat usually means that an infection is trying to enter the body, and the immune system is trying hard to defend the body. We can aid our bodies to fight off the invasion by gargling with **tea tree** (one drop to a glass of water), **lavender** or **lemon**. **Sandalwood** oil is a very powerful anti-bacterial agent, and can kill streptococci and staphylococci as effectively as most antibiotics. Whenever I have the beginnings of a sore throat, I take one drop of **sandalwood** internally. The taste is very bitter but, I think, well worth the assault on the taste buds, because one dose is usually all I need, and the sore throat does not develop into anything more serious. **Sandalwood** oil is more pleasant to take if two or three drops are added to honey water, and a teaspoonful is taken every hour or so. Not only is **sandalwood** soothing, but it has a slight analgesic quality, which takes away the 'soreness'.

Note: It is vital that the **sandalwood** oil is genuine Mysore oil, and not a **sandalwood** perfume oil, nor a **sandalwood** with added chemicals or with fatty oils to 'stretch' it, so only buy from a trustworthy company.

SHINGLES

If the immune system is below par, an adult who has not previously been exposed to the chicken pox virus can easily catch it from children. The manifestation may not be that of chicken pox but that of shingles - and in an adult this can be even more painful and distressing than the chicken pox of childhood. The chicken pox virus may even have been dormant in the body and takes hold when the immune system was at a low ebb. A homoeopathic remedy should be sought, and the affected area bathed with very dilute **lavender** or **peppermint** water. It is important that the immune system be boosted back to normal levels, and one of the ways would be to take regular aromatic baths.

Mouth Wash

Bad breath is something that can occur from a variety of causes. Perhaps we have eaten spicy or strong-tasting foods. Or were too busy to eat a meal and just drank coffee instead. Persistent worry; illness; constipation; nervousness before an event - all these things and more can make us self-conscious about our breath. There are lots of mouth washes and mouth sprays available but they all have one thing in common - they are not natural. A mouth wash can be made in the same way as a floral water for the skin, except that the mouth wash can be stronger. Several oils may be used which taste pleasant and will kill bacteria. They may be used singly or in combinations of two or three. Some of the most effective oils to use are **peppermint**; **lemon**; **lavender**; **clary sage**; **tea tree**; **bergamot**; **niaouli** and **rose**. An aromatic mouth wash will last for several weeks if kept in a dark, well stoppered bottle. (See recipe section.)

Chapter Six

Aromatherapy and the Immune System

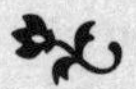

Since publication of the first edition of this book in 1985, so much information has come to light on the workings of the immune system and its significant role in our state of health, and so exciting has my own personal research been in this area that I have dedicated a whole chapter to our 'best friend', the immune system.

A great number of diseases and viruses lie dormant in our bodies, and it is not until the immune system is low, that these diseases manifest themselves. Many of the health problems in Chapter 5 are a direct result of having a weakened immune system, so allowing the disease or infection to take a hold.

Candida albicans (thrush) is a very common problem in Europe and the USA, because of the high consumption of sugar in our diets and the widespread use of antibiotics, both in medication and in the meat of animals consumed. One course of strong antibiotics can disturb the balance of the bowel flora to such an extent, that the ratio of 70 per cent friendly bacillus to 30 per cent non-friendly bacillus in the gut, can be reversed so that 70 per cent of the bacteria is harmful. As this delicate balance is responsible for the efficient functioning of our immune system, which protects us from viral, bacterial and fungal infection, it is easy to see why the problem of candida has reached epidemic proportion. The orthodox treatment for candida is a course of Nystan antibiotics, which does rather seem like 'fighting fire with fire', because although it sometimes lessens the problem over a period of weeks or months, it does not bring about a 'cure' and it subjects the body to lengthy periods of antibiotics, which further lessen the body's ability to cope with fungal infection. There are several essential oils which may be used in a douche for the treatment of vaginal

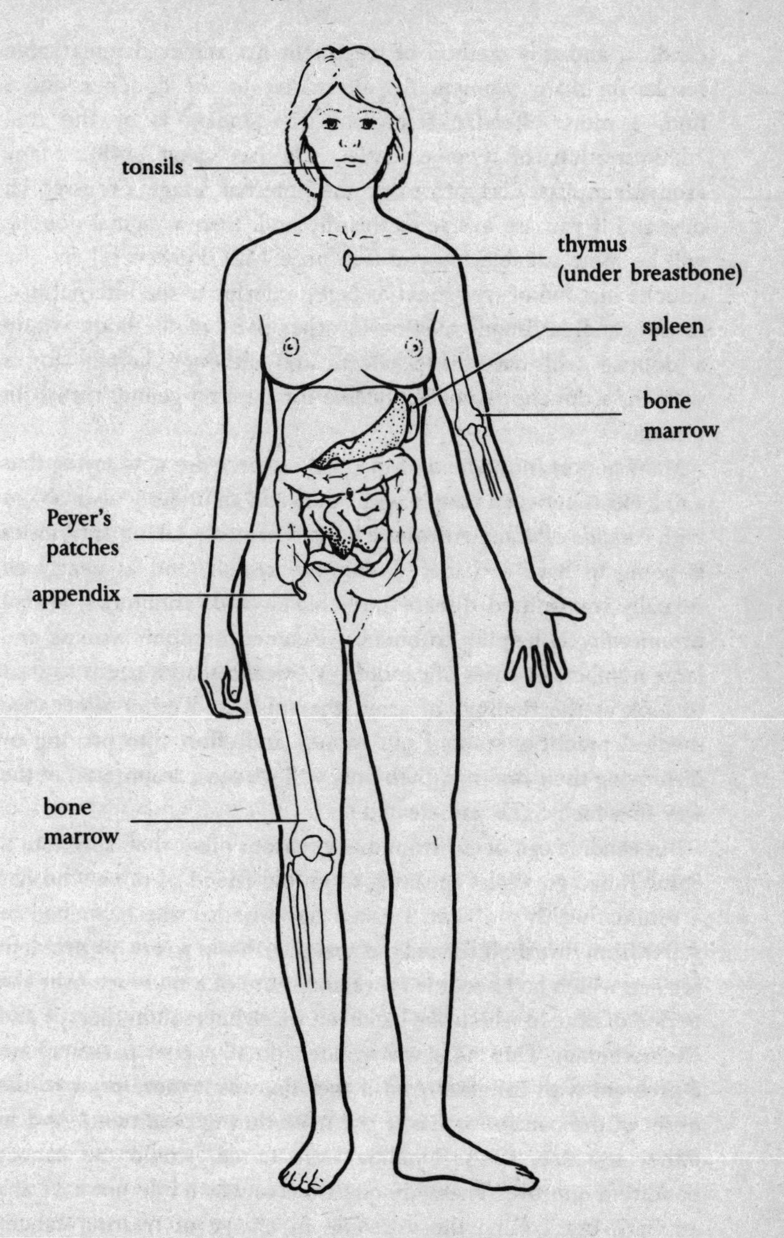

Organs of the immune system (Lymph nodes not shown)

candida, and this method of treatment has achieved remarkable results on many women. An alternative to the douches, and I find, a more effective treatment for candida is by the oral administration of two essential oils (see page 148). Many aromatherapists disapprove of the internal usage of essential oils, and if you are averse to this method, then a vaginal douche will be most suitable for you (see page 142). However, I see the douche method of treatment as being inferior to the internal use, as the candida fungus may be in other parts of the body, where a douche will have little effect, and although helpful for a woman, a douche is not applicable for treating genital thrush in a man.

Many people in the field of medical research are now saying that a link exists between people with AIDS and an underlying problem with *candida albicans*. Anyone who is repeatedly taking antibiotics is going to have a damaged immune system, and as nearly all sexually transmitted diseases are treated with antibiotics, sexual promiscuity is helping to create weakened immune systems and large numbers of cases of candida. Medical research needs to start to look at the findings of aromatherapists and other alternative medical practitioners and put money and effort into proving or disproving their findings, then only will we see a reappraisal of the way in which STDs are treated.

But candida can occur from many reasons other than antibiotics. Some time ago whilst speaking to an old friend of mine who has a serious health problem, I asked her whether she happened to suffer from thrush. It turned out that thrush was a very big problem for her, which had become more and more of a nuisance over the period of time in which she had been receiving radium therapy and chemotherapy. This made me wonder: do all cancer patients have a problem with candida? And if they do, was it there prior to the onset of the cancer, or has it occurred during treatment? And in either instance, if the candida were cured, would the cancer condition improve? These are questions to which I do not have any answers, but I hope those people in charge of treating cancer patients in oncology departments all around Britain will look eventually into the relationship between cancer, *candida albicans* and a healthy immune system.

AROMATHERAPY AND THE IMMUNE SYSTEM

Occupational stresses are responsible for weakening the immune system, and it is a well-known fact that in this age of technology, it is computer screens which are responsible for many illnesses. I recently experienced this for myself. Whilst sitting for many hours each day in front of my computer, writing a book, I was aware that one side of my face felt as though I were sitting in front of a fire. I also noticed that certain areas of my body became sensitive to touch. These areas were the glands under my jawbone, and the upper part of the breastbone. I found that by rubbing **jojoba** and **lavender** into my face, my skin was protected to some degree from the computer emissions. I also massaged the same combination into the upper chest area, paying particular attention to the sore spots. I felt that my immune system was under attack from my computer, and that my body was painful in those areas where the white blood cells were fighting to keep me healthy. It is possible to stimulate the production of white blood cells just by massaging the area above the thymus, and when this area is sensitive to touch, it needs some help from aromatherapy. Massaging this area for a few minutes, two or three times a day, will help our immune systems to help us.

In the UK more people die each year as a result of prescribed drugs than die in road traffic accidents. If these numbers of people are actually dying from prescribed drugs, how many more are suffering ill-health and damaged immune systems due to the prescribing of allopathic drugs?

Drugs are, of course, only one thing which lowers the immune system, other factors include: antibiotics; stress; VDUs; excess sugar; stimulants such as coffee and alcohol; foods which are allergens; consistent negative thinking; certain occupational hazards; overuse of sunbeds; faulty nutrition; trauma; obesity; emotional loss; saturated and unsaturated oils (in large amounts); starvation diets.

Even watching television for hours at a time is likely to result in a lowered immune system because of the radiation emitted from the screen, coupled with the content of some programmes which causes our bodies to produce adrenalin which we do not respond to (we neither fight nor run away) but merely sit and look, totally unable to help, whether it be a news bulletin or a violent detective story.

A link has been drawn between the nervous system and the immune system, and therefore those suffering from a skin condition such as eczema, where there is constant itching and scratching is continually assaulting their nervous system which in turn will adversely affect the immune system, leaving them more open to infections. Long-term benefit will be obtained from bathing in the soothing essence of **lavender** and other essential oils. Homoeopathic help should also be sought to clear up the skin condition.

Things which Strengthen the Immune System

Massage; nutritious food; love; vitamin C; zinc; positive thoughts; spiritual openness; reflexology; and of course, essential oils.

This list is by no means conclusive, but serves to give an overall picture of the diverse means of weakening or strengthening the immune system.

The immune system is incredibly complex and sophisticated. It is also known as the lymphatic system.

B cells are produced in the bone marrow (inside the long bones of the arms and legs) and *T cells* are produced in the thymus gland (situated under the breastbone). These production centres are known as *primary centres.* Other important sites of the body (tonsils; lymph nodes in the armpit; spleen; etc) are known as secondary centres. T-cells are divided into T-killers; T-helpers; and T-suppressors, and need to work with one another. The lymphocytes produced in the bone marrow are responsible for producing antibodies to any invading antigen.

Maybe we can never fully understand the immune system, but I know that we can work with it, to protect ourselves and to remain healthy and strong. The phrase 'complementary medicine' was coined to insinuate that gentle therapies, such as aromatherapy, were complementary to allopathic medicine, but as I do not like allopathic drugs, I prefer to think of the word 'complementary medicine' as meaning the gentle therapies working 'in complement' with the most incredible system of medicine - that which is going on inside us every day.

It was after reading how it is often the common illnesses such as a cold which finally kill a person with AIDS, that I thought back to the time in 1975 when my son was desperately ill. He was one year old, allergic to dairy products and had severe eczema, and had to undergo many hospital tests until a soya bean milk formula was found to be satisfactory, and he began to regain weight. After his five-week stay in hospital, I took him to a 'mother and toddler' group because I thought he needed the mental stimulus of being with other children. At that time I did not understand about the immune system, and how depleted his had become. One of the other toddlers at the group had a runny nose, but was otherwise fine. Within a short time after this encounter, my son became extremely ill. Instead of developing a cold as one would have expected, he developed severe herpes simplex, with pustular lesions in his mouth and a lesion in one of his eyes. His weakened immune system had simply been overwhelmed. He was again admitted to hospital where I was told that (as it was a viral infection) there was no medicine which would help him, and that he would have to fight it himself. I appointed myself as his intensive care nurse, and stayed by his side for two weeks, with my small collection of essences. His mouth was constantly discharging pus, and I had to lay his face on a disposable nappy which was renewed every hour or so. I swabbed the inside of his mouth with a dilute **lavender** solution, and when his temperature rose too high, I used **eucalyptus** foot compresses to reduce his fever. I also kept the atmosphere of his cubicle scented with cleansing herbal essences. In just over a week the worst of the crisis was over, and he was able to drink from a bottle again, instead of being fed via a nasal-stomach tube. The **lavender** water had cleansed, disinfected and

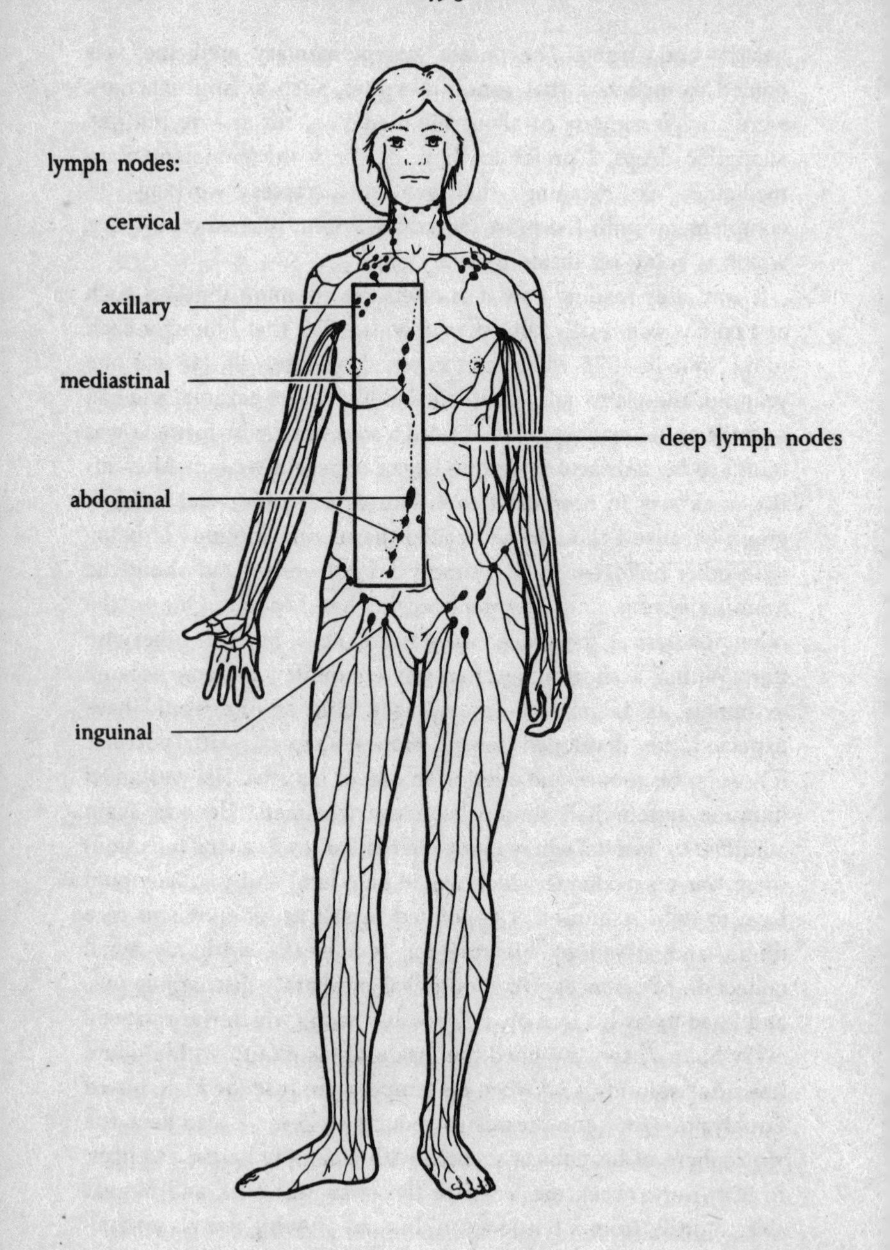

Principal groups of lymph nodes

healed the herpes lesions in the mouth, the **eucalyptus** had reduced his high temperature, and his body had been able to recharge itself, so that within a fortnight I was able to take him home.

Looking back at how a simple illness like a cold virus (herpes simplex virus) almost took the life of my son, makes me see a correlation between his situation and that of a person with AIDS. I am *not* saying here that I believe aromatherapy to be a cure for AIDS (although it might be). What I am saying is that, using the example of my son, it was he who had to regain strength and whose immune system had to rebuild its power, but whilst that was happening, it was the essences of **lavender** and **eucalyptus** which helped him to survive. Unlike antibiotics (even if they had any power over viruses) essential oils directly fight the virus or bacterial infection, encourage the body's recuperative powers and at no time compromise the immune system.

Aromatherapy has another role to play in the health of the immune system, and that is by removing the everyday stresses and negativity which weaken the immune system. If we are carrying heavy suitcases then it is not easy to walk up a hill, but if we can put them down then the climb to the top is so much easier. By removing a heavy burden from ourselves we make it easier for our immune systems to protect us. It is rather like piecing together the ends of a broken bone, so that the body's renewal system can produce the cells necessary to heal the break; nature does the healing from within, but we (the doctor in this instance) can assist that process by making sure that the bones are aligned. No doctor has ever healed a broken bone: he or she sets them. In the same way, I don't believe we are ever going to invent a 'cure' for AIDS or ME or even the 'common cold'. Common sense plays a big part in keeping our immune systems healthy, because it is our responsibility to keep ourselves in as healthy a state as possible and to facilitate the body's healing powers. We should be looking at the use of vitamin C whenever our level of health is lowered, and avoiding unhealthy foods such as hamburger and chips, cola drinks, white flour foods etc. Foods which are full of colourings and preservatives or are deep fried may not cause too much harm to a healthy person, but they are certainly not going to help a sick person to get better. Heating oil for frying (with the exception of olive oil) changes the molecular structure of the essential fatty acids and allows them to become 'oxidized'. These molecules are known as 'free radicals' and damage the surface of body cells, thereby causing a weakening of the immune system. Other obvious substances to avoid are cigarettes, drugs of any kind, alcohol, and coffee. The birth control pill also weakens the immune system and is something I hope my daughters never choose to take. There are other ways in which to avoid pregnancy, AND stay healthy.

As well as not *weakening* our immune systems, we can also *strengthen* our immune systems.

At the first sign of a throat infection (the throat is the first line of defence) gargle with **tea tree** oil or **bergamot**, in pure water.

A gargle is a sensible precaution to take after coming in contact with germs (i.e. crowds of people; travelling on planes; tube trains; sitting in doctors' waiting rooms; etc). People often wake up in the morning with a sore throat. This is because there has been a battle going on whilst they were asleep, between the body's defence system and the collection of bacteria and viruses which have entered the throat during the day.

Before going to bed for the night, a gargle with **tea tree** or one of the other recommended essences, will destroy many of the 'germs' lurking at the back of the throat, thereby helping our body's lymph glands to fight infection.

Rubbing dilute essences into the neck glands at the onset of any illness, whether a cold, flu, or something potentially more sinister, will cut short the illness by helping the immune system to fight. (See recipe on page 148.)

You should also tackle health problems as and when they occur, rather than waiting until they become huge problems which are presented to a doctor for a 'cure'. It is easy to accept a low standard of health, and to 'put up with' something like vaginal thrush, for years on end. It's easy to say, 'I get one cold after another' or, 'My son always has a runny nose.' Why do we turn a blind eye when all the clues are pointing to the fact that something is wrong? It may be an item of food which is causing an allergic reaction, or maybe the body just doesn't have the reserves of strength to wipe out the invading organisms.

We must not forget the important part that our skin has to play in the health of our body. Our skin is a living organ, the largest in our body, and it does more than just keep the rain out. By taking regular aromatherapy baths, we are repeatedly exposing our skin to small amounts of essential oils, which will not only be beneficial to the skin, but will help to strengthen the immune system. Care of the skin, massage, and cleansing of the skin are all ways in which aromatherapy will help to protect us from ill-health.

We must take responsibility for our own health, and as mothers, we need to take responsibility for the health of our children. We are the masters of our own fate. Aromatherapy and the immune system are just part of the overall picture of 'preventive medicine'.

Chapter Seven

SKIN AND HAIR CARE

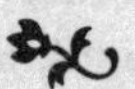

Your face may not be your fortune, but a glowing, healthy skin is the basis for looking beautiful. Many women hide under their make-up and will not be seen without it, but make-up is just another form of dressing up, and when the clothes and make-up are removed at night, we are in our natural state, with nothing left to hide behind. Very often we treat our bodies as dummies on which to hang our clothes, and apply make-up without giving much care to the condition of the skin underneath. Our skin is a living, breathing organ which is our friend and protector and deserves to be respected and well cared for. It is not mere vanity to care for and be proud of healthy, smooth skin: just good common sense.

It does not take a lot of time or a great deal of money to have a complexion that looks good, is free from blemishes and soft to the touch. All that is required is daily attention to cleansing and nourishing the skin. Nature's repair process is slow and steady, with cells being constantly renewed. This renewal of cells happens very fast in babies and children, and begins to slow down as we get older. Slower cell renewal means that skin becomes drier, allowing wrinkles to appear, dead skin cells are shed more slowly and therefore making the skin lose its youthful bloom. By using a nightly aromatherapy facial massage oil, we can cause the skin cells to renew themselves more frequently, thereby emulating the process of nature in a young person. The removal of dead skin cells, by thorough cleansing and toning of the skin each day, will also create a younger-looking skin. It is the reflection of light from the skin which denotes a youthful bloom, and conversely, it is the accumulation of dead skin cells on an older skin which prevents this reflection of light, thereby giving the appearance of dull, aged skin.

Next to smooth skin, a smile is your best asset, lighting up the face of the 'plainest of Janes'. So soothe away the cares of the day in aromatic baths; sprinkle essences around your home and office; and try to sort out little health problems before they become a worry.

Real beauty comes from within. It is not something we can buy in pots, massage in, or obtain from a beauty salon. But it is something that can be acquired, as a whole person improves her state of health, vitality and confidence. We don't have to accept what we see in the mirror, because if we don't like it we can change it. I don't mean by plastic surgery, because I don't think that wrinkles or a large nose make any difference to a person's beauty. Beauty comes from within and everyone has the power to possess healthy shining hair, sparkling eyes, satin-smooth skin, and a happy countenance. For me meditation is vitally important for my well-being and happiness, and has caused a beautiful transformation in my life. But with or without a spiritual anchor, we can improve upon how we look, and continuously care for the skin with aromatherapy, a good diet, and a positive attitude to life.

To me, the human body is like a car which takes us from A to B, and we are the owner of that car. Either we can look after the vehicle and be a proud owner, or leave it to get rusty and fall apart, bit by bit. If the car is neglected for a long time, it will require much effort and patience to restore it to peak condition. But if it is cared for and attended to regularly, it will continue to be of service indefinitely.

According to a survey carried out in the USA, the thing that men found most exciting and attractive about a woman was not her face, or legs, or bosom, but the way she felt about herself, which was reflected in the way she carried herself. That is the sex appeal that we all have. We all have an ideal of how we would like to look or admire someone beautiful, but we can never look like the person, any more than we could change our fingerprints. We are all unique and special in our own way, and it is from that basic understanding that we are as wretched or as beautiful as we experience ourselves to be. Marilyn Monroe, the idol of millions, was unhappy about her nose! Few of us are born as beautiful as Monroe, but all of us can improve ourselves and realize our full potential. The part of us which is unseen is far more beautiful than the part which is seen.

USING ESSENTIAL OILS ON THE SKIN

Essential oils are very powerful substances, and must be handled with respect. Certain essential oils should never be used on the skin, and these oils are either omitted from this book or, when they have been used medicinally, they are accompanied by a warning that they should not be used on the skin (e.g. **clove** oil).

Essential oils are safe to use on the skin, providing that the following points are remembered:

- Ensure that you are using true essential oils, and not a 'perfume' labelled as an essential oil. Always buy your essential oils from a reputable company that you know you can trust. Even high street shops do not always offer pure oils - ask them if they can really vouch for the purity of the essential oils on sale.
- Never use neat essential oils on the face (with the exception of dabbing spots with **lavender** or **tea tree**). Apart from being too concentrated, a fatty oil is necessary in order to disperse the essences and to provide 'spreadability' for a massage.
- Don't use mineral oil (such as baby oil) with essential oils, as mineral oil will not penetrate the skin, and will inhibit the action of the essential oils. (Mineral oil acts as a skin barrier, which is the reason it is so widely used for coating babies' bottoms.)
- Dilute essential oils in a carrier oil. Use any of the vegetable oils or nut oils such as **sweet almond**, **camellia**, **apricot kernel**, **sunflower**,

hazelnut etc. Even **olive** oil may be used, but it has a strong aroma of its own, and I find that it overpowers the more delicate aromas.
Wheatgerm oil contains natural vitamin E (which is an anti-oxidant), and I like to add 10 per cent **wheatgerm** oil to a massage oil if I intend to keep it for more than a week. Massage blends which are intended for use within a day or so of making them need not include the **wheatgerm** oil. People with coeliac disease cannot tolerate **wheatgerm** oil, and therefore a fresh massage oil should be prepared.

- For a daily facial massage oil, a blend consisting of 98 per cent base oil to 2 per cent essential oil is ideal (see pages 149-50).
- If your hand should accidentally slip whilst adding drops of essential oil to the base oil, and more essence has been added than you intended, simply increase the amount of base oil.
- Essential oils do not dissolve in water, but will disperse sufficiently to be used for cleansing the skin if the mixture is shaken thoroughly. The mixture should be shaken well before use.

How Essential Oils Work Through the Skin

The beauty of an aromatherapy facial massage is that it is not just working on the surface of the skin, but is a real treatment which works on a deeper level. Essential oils, because of their volatile nature, have the ability to penetrate through the skin to the dermis, the underlying layers of the skin. Essential oils also travel through the interstitial fluid, the bloodstream and the lymphatic system.

It is possible to effect a remarkable change in the condition of the skin by applying a treatment oil each night before going to bed. Apply the blend with a gentle massage, using light, upward strokes, and leave it to work whilst you are asleep. In this simple way, a flawless complexion can be acquired and then maintained.

Whichever skin type we have, the same sequence of events can be used: thorough cleansing at night, followed by an aromatherapy facial massage oil.

I have not bought any commercial skin care products for almost 20 years, preferring to mix up my own. The cleansing of the skin is very important, and I use a floral water to take off my make-up, and the dirt of the day. Some mascaras will not come off in this way, and then I find that a small amount of **jojoba** is the perfect answer. It will remove every last trace of mascara without putting strain on the delicate tissues around the eyes. **Jojoba** is also beneficial to the eyelashes, and may even repair lashes which have been damaged by the overuse of eye make-up. In the early seventies I wore false eyelashes, as was the fashion, and my natural eyelashes suffered as a consequence. I cannot say categorically that **jojoba** will make your eyelashes grow thicker and longer, but there should be a noticeable improvement as there has been with mine. After removing the **jojoba** residues and make-up particles with a cotton wool ball dipped into floral water, your face is ready for the facial massage.

Oily/Acneic Skin

Nothing could be more perfect than aromatherapy for treating oily and acneic complexions, as essences have an affinity with the skin, being able to pass through the skin barrier via the fluids and penetrate into the body. Many essential oils are cleansing and anti-bacterial; for example **lavender, bergamot, neroli, sandalwood, tea tree, ylang-ylang, ravansara** and **lemon**, and these will help us to correct a skin which is infected with acne and teenage spots. Hormonal changes during puberty cause the body to produce substances which, if not eliminated via the kidneys and liver, will build up and cause eruptions on the face and neck and occasionally on other parts of the body. Antibiotics are routinely prescribed for this condition, but it seems to me to be adding fuel to the fire. If the body is not eliminating properly, then it seems senseless to overburden it with drugs which have to pass through the kidneys, and are therefore creating more of a toxic problem. It makes more sense to detoxify the entire body, using a combination of good diet, blood purifying tablets*, and essential oil massage and baths. The temptation to apply astringents or to squeeze spots should be avoided, as these methods will not cure the condition and will only stimulate the sebaceous glands to work overtime and encourage the spread of bacteria.

A nightly facial massage with a blend for acne (see recipe on page 149) will work on a deep level, imparting a natural antiseptic to the infected areas, and at the same time regulating the secretion of sebum.

Thorough cleansing of the skin is important, and a herbal cleansing water (see recipe on page 150) will remove most make-up and surface dirt from the skin, and if rough cotton wool is used for a second application, the action will be similar to that of an exfoliant - that is, the dead skin cells will be removed, leaving the skin looking fresh and radiant. After thorough cleansing, a liberal amount of 'acne blend' should be applied to the face and neck and massaged into the skin in upward sweeps. Tissue off any excess oil after a few minutes by placing a tissue over the skin, and blotting gently. Very toxic skins will not absorb much oil but, when used regularly over a period of time, the skin's improvement will be indicated by its ability to absorb more oil. Do not expect a flawless complexion overnight, but treat your skin each day and soon you will begin to notice a difference in appearance and texture.

DRY SKIN

A hot climate, illness, central heating or bad diet can all affect the skin, causing it to feel and look dry and taut. Dry skin, because

* Echinacea tablets are available from health food stores, and are wonderful blood purifiers.

of a lack of natural oils, becomes wrinkled more easily than greasy skin, and needs daily 'feeding' with protective and nourishing oils. A special blend of essential oils, chosen for their ability to improve the condition of dry skin (see recipe on page 150) should be gently massaged into the face and neck every night before going to bed. Before the facial massage, the skin may be gently cleansed with one of the floral waters, and in the mornings you can create your own 'moisturizer' by leaving a fine layer of floral water on your skin, before lightly applying a tiny amount of massage oil. Dry skin will soak up these blends, but before applying make-up, blot the face with a tissue to remove any excess oils. Dryness of the skin can also be caused by living in centrally-heated homes and offices; overuse of sunbeds; an imbalance of vitamins and minerals; by hormonal changes during the menopause; stress; smoking and other pollutants. Improving the condition of your environment will help to maintain your improved skin tone and texture, and the use of a humidifier or ionizer in homes and offices should be considered.

Mature Skin

As we grow older our skin cells do not renew themselves quite as quickly as they did when we were young, which is why the skin loses its soft bloom and elasticity, forming wrinkles and lines. Some essential oils could rightly be called rejuvenators, because they have the capability of speeding up the re-growth of skin cells, thereby preserving a youthful looking skin which is healthy and soft to the touch. Rejuvenation is a word which is forbidden to be used in advertising in the UK, yet that is precisely what essential oils do. Some essences, such as **lavender**, have the ability to encourage the growth of new skin cells - this is illustrated by the experience of one of my friends. She had burnt her hand, and although the burn had healed and was no longer painful, a visible scar remained on the skin for several months. Various creams and ointments were tried, but nothing removed the scar, until neat **lavender** oil was applied. Within a very short space of time, the scar had disappeared completely.

Other essential oils which fall into the category of rejuvenators are: **neroli, rose, myrrh** and **frankincense**. A massage oil should be made up (see recipe on page 150) and the face and neck massaged every night. Essential oils work on the underlying tissues whilst you are sleeping, and if used regularly, a marked improvement will be noticed.

To aid penetration of the massage oil, and to make you feel cosseted and pampered, apply a **neroli** facial compress (see page 151) after your facial massage and then lie down for half an hour or so, with your favourite music in the background.

FLORAL WATERS

A limited selection of floral waters are available commercially, but many contain either synthetic aromas or alcohol, neither of which is good for the skin. Making your own aromatic waters is very cost effective and much more fun. Essential oils are natural cleansers, and so these floral waters are ideal for cleansing your face at the end of the day. Mascara and other eye make-up may not be removed by a watery solution, but a little **jojoba** oil on cotton wool will do the job beautifully. **Jojoba** is also beneficial to the eyelashes, strengthening and thickening them. Remove the excess **jojoba** oil with the floral water. A beautifully clean face for a few pence! Alcohol is often used in commercial toners and floral waters, but it is bad for the skin and will make dry skin even drier. I do not like tap water as it contains a whole host of chemicals which I prefer not to put on my skin. To use a bottled spa water whenever possible is more economical in the long run, because the floral water will 'keep' for a longer period of time. Tap water may be used but because it contains bacteria it will not 'keep' for long and should be discarded as soon as the aroma alters, and a fresh solution made up. The other disadvantage of using tap water is the fact that it contains chlorine and heavy metals. It has become popular to purchase mineral water sprays for use on the face, and although delightfully refreshing on a hot day, or after strenuous exercise, they do work out rather expensive. I have an aversion to aerosol sprays so prefer to make a floral water with my choice of essence in mineral water, and then add it to a clean empty mist spray bottle. Spray your face (even over make-up) when in any situation which could cause the skin to dehydrate, such as whilst flying long distances, or being out of doors for long periods during hot weather.

I like to use a **clary sage** floral water in the mornings, as the aroma makes me feel cheerful and ready to start the day. Then at night-time I use a **lavender** floral water to remove make-up and prepare me for a restful sleep.

Facial Masks

Every now and again it is beneficial to have a facial mask, which will draw impurities to the surface of the skin and stimulate circulation. There are a great many available in the shops, but it is fun and very much more economical to make one's own (see recipe on page 151). If your skin is very greasy, you may safely leave the mask on until it dries; however, if you have dry skin, the mask should be removed after 5-10 minutes. To remove the mask, just soak cotton wool in warm water and wipe over the face, taking off the clay, and continue to use fresh pieces of cotton wool until the face is clean. When all traces of the mask have been removed, gently swab the skin with cotton wool soaked in floral water and finally apply a little facial massage oil to the skin, or alternatively, pat on a little '**rose** body perfume'.

Facial masks should not be used too frequently as they will draw out not only impurities from the skin, but also the skin's natural oils, and overuse will cause dry skin to become even drier. Probably the optimum frequency of use is once a month.

Eye Compress

Tired eyes, or those irritated by contact lenses or a smoky atmosphere, will find immediate relief from a **neroli, camomile** or **lavender** eye compress. Add one drop of essence into a 500ml bottle of spring water and shake well. After soaking two cotton wool pads in the liquid, squeeze out excess water and place a pad over each eye.

Crying is very beneficial and can release a lot of stored tensions and emotions. A good cry can be akin to spring cleaning your house, but although you might feel a great sense of relief afterwards, one look in the mirror can be rather disheartening. Puffy red eyes can be soothed and made to regain their normal appearance quickly by applying a **lavender** or **camomile** compress to each eye. Use a piece of cotton wool about the size of the palm of your hand (so that the compress is large enough not only to cover the immediate eye area but also to treat any puffiness to the upper cheeks and the area up to and including the eyebrows). If possible, lie down for half an hour with some soothing music playing in the background.

Note: Always remove contact lenses before using an eye compress.

Rose Rub

Keep your body looking great and smelling divine by treating it to the therapeutic powers of **rose** (see recipe on page 150). After bathing, rub a little into the skin of the face and body, paying particular attention to parts of the body which tend towards dryness and are looking aged. It is said that one can tell the age of a woman by her elbows as this part of the anatomy has very little body fat overlying the bone and therefore becomes dry and wrinkled very easily, but with the help of **jojoba** and **rose** oil massaged firmly into the area all around the elbows, I think it may be possible to 'take off' a few years.

Jojoba Oil

Jojoba oil was used by the Native American Indians for many skin complaints, as well as for treating both dry and greasy skins, and for protecting and conditioning their hair, and would have been a prized commodity. The Native Americans did not have the choice of products that you or I have, but I think they were very fortunate to have the **jojoba**, and even though I have a vast choice, **jojoba** is a firm favourite of mine, which I would not like to be without. Because **jojoba** is such a wonderful emollient it is playing its part in conservation, being used instead to spermaceti, which means that the whale population of the world is no longer being hunted to extinction. Many are the properties of **jojoba**, some of which are unique. Its uniqueness may owe something to the fact that the **jojoba** bush grows in arid deserts of North America, where nothing else will grow. It survives by sending a tap root as much as 40 feet down into the ground to obtain moisture, and halts its own growth when there is a lack of vital nutrients in the soil. **Jojoba** contains traces of iodine and proteins, and because it is a liquid wax, it will solidify when placed in a refrigerator. My experience with **jojoba** shows that it has the ability to emulsify fat, and tone the tissues, making it ideal to use whilst dieting or losing weight through exercising. **Jojoba** protects the skin, and therefore makes an ideal barrier for the hands, as well as for babies' bottoms to guard against nappy rash. **Jojoba** is thought to be anti-allergenic, which means that even the most sensitive of skins will be able to tolerate it.

Jojoba has been referred to throughout this book, but nowhere more so than in this chapter, as I find it quite indispensable for skin and hair care.

Hair Rinses

Several essential oils are traditionally used as a final rinsing water for each of the different hair types. It is difficult to buy shampoos which are natural, although some are more natural than others, but a beautiful and natural fragrance can be added to your hair, by rinsing the hair with an aromatic water. Commonly used rinses are **rosemary** and **camomile**. **Rosemary** is traditionally recommended to bring lustre and depth to dark hair.

Camomile is the herb recommended for blonde hair, as it has a natural lightening effect on fair hair. But why not try a really exotic hair rinse, when you want to smell absolutely divine! **Rose**, although expensive, is unsurpassable, and will make your hair smell as though you have stepped out of the pages of a fairytale - as a princess attending the ball and turning all heads. Or rinse your hair with **frankincense**, for those times when you want to feel spiritually uplifted. Rinses can be made up and stored in a brown bottle (available from chemists) or use an empty wine bottle with a well-fitting cork. (See page 152).

Almost any essence can be used as a hair rinse, but whichever essence is used, it must be thoroughly shaken in a bottle of water before use. **Patchouli** oil is dark and heavy but, when one drop is mixed well in water, will bring a soft sensuous aroma to dark hair - to me it is very reminiscent of the late sixties and of my search for truth. Almost any essential oil could be used as a final rinse for the hair, and you could change the rinse according to the perfume you were going to wear or to the mood which you wanted to create.

Treatment for Damaged Hair

Hair can be damaged by many different things: the weather, perming, colouring, crimping, bleaching, or even by frequent washing with a strong shampoo. Whatever the reason for damage, if your hair is lacking in lustre and is feeling dry, then a once-a-week oil treatment will replace vital nutrients, making the hair look better, at the same time as feeding the scalp and improving the 'soil' in which the hair grows.

You will need to set aside two to three hours. Firstly (after making up one of the blends on page 152) part the hair into sections, pour some of the treatment oil into a saucer or small bowl, and dip in a piece of cotton wool. Apply the mixture along the parting, and continue to section the hair in this way until the entire head has been completed. Then stroke the oil-soaked cotton wool all the way down to the end of your hair. Because the very end of the hair is the most prone to be dry and split, make sure that you are generous with the treatment oil in this area. When all the hair has been saturated, pile it on top of the head and wrap it in a towel. A minimum of two hours should elapse before you wash the hair, to ensure that the oil has the chance to work thoroughly. It is best to firstly work in some shampoo and a small amount of water, in order to create an emulsion, and after washing this away to proceed to wash your hair as normal.

Treatment for Greasy Hair

Greasy hair is the result of overactive sebaceous glands, which is quite a common occurrence during puberty, at the time of the monthly period, and during times of stress. Certain essential oils have a normalizing effect on the sebaceous glands, but without being astringent and drying up the scalp. **Tea tree** oil, **lemon**, **geranium** and **lavender** are some of the oils which would be beneficial for tackling the problem of greasy hair, and at the same time will safeguard against pimples on the scalp, as these essences are anti-bacterial. The essential oils should be massaged gently into the scalp, after first mixing up the formulation for greasy hair (see recipe on page 151). Once the recipe has been made up, proceed as for treatment of damaged hair.

Treatment for Head Lice

Head lice used to be a problem when ladies wore wigs and rarely washed their hair, and this is understandable, but today we find that there is a recurrence of the age-old problem even though women now wash their hair more frequently than at any time in the past. The reasons for this phenomenon are open to discussion, but perhaps as the infestation rate in schools is so high the problem is also reaching adults and being transferred that way. Lice have now become resistant to certain chemicals which would once have been fatal to them. They also seem to have become more tenacious. Lice can remain alive for more than 10 hours just by clinging to a single strand of hair, and it really is unwise to borrow another person's hairbrush. Head lice seem to survive for long periods of time under water, and no matter how much swimming, diving, showering and hair washing one does, it is almost impossible to drown them. The only way to kill lice seems to be by using either a chemical or essential oils, to which the lice have no tolerance. Of the many 'lice mixtures' on sale in chemists some are alcohol-based, and these can sometimes cause scalp irritation, and as heat and alcohol is a dangerous combination, the hair must be left to dry naturally. If you have long hair and are unlucky enough to get lice, then this could take all day. Using the combination of essential oils to combat the problem will not only kill the lice within two hours, but will cost a fraction of the price of a chemist-preparation, and will leave your hair healthy and lustrous.

Make up the recipe on page 152 and section the hair, carefully applying the mixture to the hair roots and scalp. Stroke the mixture through the rest of the hair, and pile it on top of your head, wrapping a long sheet of clingfilm carefully around your head to ensure that all the hair is securely trapped inside. This is a little difficult to do by yourself, and if you cannot get a helping hand, I would recommend that you remove the clingfilm from its cardboard dispenser, and wrap the film around the head going over the ears, gradually working towards the centre of your head. When all of your hair is covered by clingfilm, you can tuck the plastic behind your ears.

TREATMENT FOR DANDRUFF

Dandruff occurs when there is an imbalance of oils at the skin's surface, and although one may suppose that it is a problem associated with dry skin, it tends to occur as a result of overactive sebaceous glands, and often affects those people who have acne. Although not harmful, dandruff is an embarrassment, when there is noticeable dead skin littering the shoulders, and when particles of dead skin adhere to greasy hair strands. Dandruff can also occur as a result of a person eating foods to which he or she is allergic, or when suffering from *candida albicans.* For example, my eldest daughter, at the age of 9 months, developed very severe cradle cap, which coincided with the introduction of dairy products into her diet. Over the years I have tried to steer her away from milk foods but as she does not have any other symptoms, I have not insisted on her being vegan like her brother. However, I can always tell when she has binged on pizzas or milkshakes because of the condition of her scalp, and the appearance of dandruff.

Dandruff should act as a warning that there is a problem, of whatever size, and steps should be taken to find out why the scalp is unhealthy. If dandruff is accompanied by regular headaches or a stiff neck, it is possible that there is a subluxation of the cervical bones in the neck, which a visit to a chiropractor could rectify. But a topical treatment, based on **jojoba** and **tea tree** oil, will greatly improve the condition of the scalp, and lessen the shedding of skin onto the shoulders. The best essential oil for dandruff is Australian **tea tree** oil, which smells a little like **eucalyptus**, but is much more gentle on the skin. Its anti-bacterial and anti-fungal properties prevent the development of any secondary infections whilst dealing quickly and safely with the problem of seborrhoea. As mentioned in an earlier chapter, **tea tree** is very safe on the skin, but a very small percentage of people (such as my son) cannot tolerate it. If you have very sensitive skin, it is therefore advisable to apply a little **tea tree** oil to a small area of the forearm before treating the entire scalp. I have blended together **jojoba** and **tea tree**, as each has healing properties which will help to alleviate dandruff, but for those people who do not like the smell of **tea tree**, or are sensitive to it, **jojoba** may be used on its own. **Jojoba** oil is one of the best products of nature for treating dandruff, and should be massaged into the scalp two or three times a week.

Make up a recipe from page 151 and proceed as for 'damaged hair'.

Conditioner for Normal Hair

To impart an incredible shine to normal hair, take some good quality fatty oil, add **jojoba** oil and some essential oils, and massage through the hair, paying particular attention to the ends, especially on long hair, where split ends could be a problem. Arrange the hair on top of the head, and cover with a towel. Leave on for 30 minutes to one hour and then wash off, adding shampoo and a little water to first make an emulsion, before washing in the normal way with a mild shampoo. **Jojoba** oil is much more expensive than **sweet almond** and other nut oils, and only 10 per cent **jojoba** need be used in the base oil. I would always use this combination of ingredients if I had very long hair. However, as my hair is fairly short, I tend to use **jojoba** and essential oils to condition my hair, without using the nut oil base.

A once-weekly treatment will condition hair beautifully, and add a lustre that ordinary conditioners don't quite manage. An aromatherapy conditioner works in an entirely different way from the type of conditioner bought in a supermarket. Commercial conditioners are formulated to change the chemical coating of the hair, altering the molecular structure from positive to negative, and therefore are of cosmetic use only. **Jojoba** works in quite a different way, because although the liquid wax does coat the hairs, making them smooth and shiny, there is also considerable benefit done to the scalp, and a healthy scalp is the basis of having healthy, shining hair. The aroma of **jojoba** is not unpleasant, having a slightly burnt smell, but I like to improve upon the natural aroma of **jojoba**, and surround myself with fragrance whilst I am giving myself a hair and scalp conditioning treatment. Sometimes I add a drop of **rosewood**, sometimes a drop of **sandalwood**, sometimes even a drop of **rose**, but most commonly I use a drop of **clary sage**.

Chapter Eight

PREGNANCY AND CHILDBIRTH

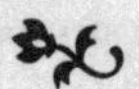

TAKING GOOD CARE OF YOURSELF

It was during my pregnancies, while indulging myself in frequent aromatic baths, and scenting the atmosphere of my home with beautiful aromas, that I noticed how much less prone I was to catching colds, or any illness for that matter. Maybe this is due to the fact that pregnancy produces extra antibodies in defence of the new life growing within, but I like to think that my extraordinarily healthful state was due in part to my aromatic lifestyle. This is not hard to imagine, when you consider that the only people said to survive the great plague of London were perfumers, glovers (who used essential oils to cure the leather) and those doctors who carried a walking stick in which the top was hollow and filled with aromatic herbs and spices.

Water is very good for pregnant women - drinking lots of mineral water, swimming regularly and, of course, relaxing aromatic baths. For an aromatic bath almost any essential oil that you really like will benefit you, and it is a matter of personal preference. I remember being particularly fond of **petitgrain** oil during my first pregnancy, and whenever I smell **petitgrain** oil it instantly reminds me of that time. **Clary sage** and **geranium** oils are both great morale boosters, especially towards the end of the pregnancy when each day seems like an eternity, and one wonders if the baby is ever going to arrive.

Lavender is a must during pregnancy, as it has the longest list of therapeutic properties, together with being the safest oil on the skin. What a piece of creative genius! Can you imagine the triumph for a pharmaceutical company which could produce one substance that could be used in the bath, on the skin, as a perfume, to bring about relaxation, promote healing, treat burns, stop bleeding, and promote restful sleep, plus many more uses. It would be impossible! In the creation of **lavender**, we can see the skill of a master perfumer, the genius of the best scientist, plus the knowledge of all cosmetic chemists rolled into one, to make a substance which is almost a medicine chest in a bottle. To say that **lavender** is beneficial during pregnancy is an understatement; it has the ability to stimulate the production of healthy white blood cells, and to goad them into action, should an invading organism, such as a cold virus, decide to visit. I would recommend a **lavender** bath at least once a week during pregnancy.

Tea tree baths are toning and will help you shake off a cold should you succumb to one. **Tea tree** has anti-fungal and anti-bacterial properties and will improve many skin conditions. It is an excellent alternative to **lavender** oil for healing burns or treating sunburn for those people who, for whatever reason, do not like the aroma of **lavender**. During the summer I find that **bergamot** or **rosewood** baths are delightfully refreshing, and can be enjoyed either in the morning or the evening. Other light, refreshing essences which make ideal bath additives are **lemon, orange, rosemary, orange blossom** and **clary sage**. Heavier and sweeter aromas are **sandalwood**, **geranium**, **rose**, **jasmine**, **patchouli** and **ylang-ylang**. **Peppermint** oil, when used sparingly, makes for a wonderfully cooling bath in the midst of summer. I was heavily pregnant during the heatwave of 1976, and **peppermint** baths saved my sanity many times. To a bath of tepid water, just add 2–4 drops of **peppermint**, mix well, slide in and defuse.

Throughout pregnancy you are a very important person. This is a time for being selfish, for taking the best care of yourself that you can. Your state of health will be reflected in your baby. Your state of mind will also have an effect on the foetus growing inside you. Whatever you eat, whatever you drink and, to a certain extent, whatever you apply to your skin, will be building blocks for the growth and formation of your child. Positive and beautiful thoughts can alter our basic cravings for things which may be harmful to the baby. Sometimes habits are hard to break, but we should try to remember that although nine months is only a short span of time out of our own lifetime, to a developing baby it is the most critical period of its entire life. It is when we feel a bit down or depressed that the temptation to reach for a glass of alcohol or a cigarette is strongest, and at these times perhaps we can reach for a safe alternative, a **clary sage** bath to lift depression, or one of the Bach Flower Remedies, for instance. I find that Rescue Remedy is extremely useful to take at stressful times, especially so after an accident, however minor.

CONSTIPATION

Constipation during pregnancy is uncomfortable, unhealthy for both the mother and the baby, and usually unnecessary if a sensible pattern of eating is followed. I was a vegetarian before any of my

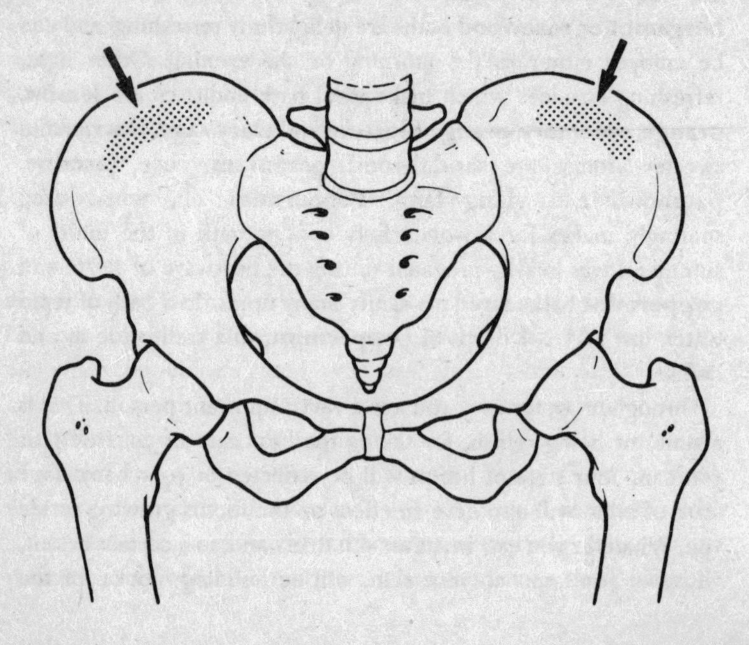

children were conceived, and as my diet was full of brown rice and salads, wholemeal bread and mineral water, I was rarely bothered by discomfort. Whether we are vegetarian, 'fishetarian' or carnivore, there are certain foods which are best avoided, or only eaten in small quantities. Cheese, too many eggs, white bread, and other white flour products will all increase the likelihood of constipation. Red meats, as they take many days to digest in the intestines, are more likely to aggravate constipation than salad vegetables, which are digested quicker. Most vegetables contain fibre, which gives the intestines something to get hold of, and so these should be eaten daily. Tension can also be a contributing factor towards constipation, and therefore relaxing baths are recommended.

For anyone who does suffer badly from constipation, I would recommend a massage of the lower back area using a simple blend of oils (see page 153). Particular attention should be given to the area at either side of the spine, within the pelvic frame (see diagram on page 104). If you can get a partner to massage this area for you be prepared for a little pain, as this area is always tender to the touch if the intestines are not functioning properly. It is possible to massage this area yourself while standing up, but don't cheat. Apply some pressure to the sore spot, in the knowledge that a little discomfort now is better than the long-term discomfort of constipation.

PURIFYING THE ATMOSPHERE

It used to be standard practice for doctors and midwives to don white facial masks before delivering the baby, but I hope this relatively pointless ritual has now been abandoned. Airborne bacteria are so tiny that they penetrate through the gauze masks as soon as the wearer speaks or coughs, so there seems little point in them being worn, unless it is for the psychological benefit of the woman in labour. However, airborne bacteria are vulnerable to essential oil vapours so, whether giving birth at home or in hospital, keep a small bowl of warm water by the bedside, to which to add your oils. Strong anti-bacterial essences should be used, preferably those with a light fragrance such as **bergamot, lemon, lavender** or **niaouli**. **Eucalyptus** could be used, or its cousin, **myrtle**, although some people would find these two oils just a little too overpowering. **Tea tree** is a wonderful antiseptic oil, although the aroma is disliked by some people. I find that **tea tree** blends well with **lavender** or **lemon**, to produce a very fresh aroma which is antiseptic but also a million times nicer than hospital disinfectant smells.

By utilizing essential oils as a room purifier, you are protecting your immediate environment from the germs and viruses which constantly surround us. I once watched a doctor and some nurses don protective garments, face masks, and gloves before entering the room in which a sick child lay, and I wanted to ask them what measures they had taken to sterilize their shoes. So small are the bugs which cause us disease, that they cannot be seen with our eyes, but how wonderful that our nose can tell us whether or not we are being protected. I find it very comforting to know that whenever I inhale essential oil vapours I am breathing in vital forces which protect and strengthen me.

Labour Massage

The pain experienced in the lower back during the hours of labour can be alleviated by massage. Provided that you have a sympathetic partner or friend willing to sit with you during labour, you will find great comfort from a firm massage to your lower back. It would be advisable to practise this during the last month of pregnancy, so that you find the position most comfortable to you, and so that you may also coach your partner to carry out the massage to your instructions. Massage itself, using firm rhythmic pressure, is a very welcome experience to a woman in labour. Blending those essential oils which can help to relieve pain and promote relaxation into a massage oil base greatly enhances the effectiveness of the massage.

Massage should be given at intervals, when the woman feels the need, and according to the stamina of the giver of the massage.

Some labours can be extremely long. My first labour was 27 hours in duration and, as I was determined to 'do it naturally' without any drugs, I'm afraid that after the birth of our son, my husband was more in need of recuperation than I was! Many women prefer to go into hospital and accept the medication on offer. My twin sister is of this opinion, and would never have dreamt of giving birth in the way that I did. We should all be able to have our babies in the place, and in the way that is comfortable to ourselves. Childbirth is not a disease, needing medical intervention; and entering the world need not be clinical and harsh, but rather gentle and mystical, so that you can fully appreciate the miracle that is taking place. Many more hospitals are offering expectant mothers the facilities to squat, give birth in dimly-lit rooms, or even in a tank of water; if the mother wants her other children to be present, this can also be arranged. This is a big improvement in the quality of hospital maternity care, but my first choice has always been to give birth to my children at home, with the care of an experienced midwife.

Pregnancy and Childbirth

Pregnancy is a time I have enjoyed tremendously. I think my enjoyment was enhanced by using essences instead of conventional treatments, and just allowing myself to delight in the process that was happening inside me. Never have I had such a good excuse for wallowing in deep warm baths whenever I felt like it. Many essential oils should be avoiding during pregnancy, and as well as the hundreds of obscure essential oils (those which are not written about in books because little or no research has been carried out) the following essences should be *avoided:* **basil**, **cinnamon**, **clove**, **hyssop**, **myrrh**, **origanum**, **pennyroyal**, **sage**, **savoury** and **thyme**.

Nausea

There is nothing safer or more effective for morning sickness than **peppermint** oil, either on brown sugar, or in honey water. Nausea is a very common problem in the early stages of pregnancy, but it is easily remedied with a sensible diet and **peppermint** oil (or even **peppermint** tea, taken several times a day if preferred). There is no necessity to seek relief with prescribed drugs, and the thalidomide tragedies would never have occurred, if doctors and antenatal classes had recommended their pregnant patients to take herb teas and essential oils, instead of inconclusively tested chemicals.

One drop of **peppermint**, taken every hour until relief is obtained is usually adequate to bring relief, but in very severe cases, where the woman constantly vomits, then it would be preferable to take a homoeopathic remedy (such as Ipecacuanha) or apply a **lavender** compress to the abdomen: add two drops of **lavender** oil to a bowl of warm water, soak a small towel in the liquid, wring it out, then apply to the abdomen. Place a larger towel over the top, and rest for 30 minutes or so.

Pregnant women are very sensitive to smells, because our sense of smell - which is often neglected - becomes more acute during pregnancy. During my pregnancies I liked to surround myself with a healthy, scented atmosphere. My favourite essences were **bergamot, geranium, lavender** and **rose**. To a bowl of hot water, I would pour a few drops of one or more of these and let the aromatic vapours fill the atmosphere. So simple and therapeutic is this action, that one day I hope to see aromatic air purifiers being used in antenatal clinics, maternity hospitals, doctors' waiting rooms, and indeed, anywhere that the public meet and where infections are readily passed from one person to another via the atmosphere. A handful of hospitals are already using essential oils in the wards, to create an uplifting and healthful atmosphere, and I am sure that by the turn of the century, this practice will become very much more widespread.

Stretch Marks

As the breasts and abdomen grow bigger and bigger, the skin has to stretch phenomenally, and unfortunately this can lead to stretch marks - tiny scars in the underlying tissues of the skin. Once formed these scars are difficult to get rid of, and prevention is better than cure. A twice daily massage with a 'pregnancy massage oil' will reduce the likelihood of stretch marks. Using light sweeping movements, gently rub the oil into the skin of the abdomen. A light massage feels delightful in itself, and I am sure the baby will like it too. A healthy diet, full of raw, energizing foods, will contribute greatly to healthy skin, which will stretch as far as it needs to, and then return to normal. Anyone who already has stretch marks from a pregnancy or through losing weight quickly during dieting, need not despair as a daily massage with **lavender** in **jojoba** and **wheatgerm** oil (see page 153) will gradually bring about an improvement.

HEARTBURN

The part of pregnancy I most hated and dreaded was the heartburn. I suffered with it for about the last six weeks of each pregnancy. When expecting my first child, I took **peppermint** oil, which had helped enormously with the earlier nausea. It helped a little, but I can remember waking up every two hours or so during the night to sip water or **peppermint** tea, just so that I could go back to sleep again. I did not want to take antacid tablets and during my second pregnancy I took some **rose** oil, and found that this gave me longer periods of heartburn-relief than the **peppermint**. However it was not perfect, and during my third pregnancy I wanted something better. My husband had discovered, in some ancient text, that **sandalwood** was good for heartburn, as it was a bitter-tasting essential oil. I took one drop, and found the taste rather unpleasant but not intolerable, and, as it worked and allowed me to sleep soundly all night, I recommend it wholeheartedly. As I could not tolerate anything sweet, I took the drop of **sandalwood** neat, and not on sugar or in honey water, as is normally the best method.

Note: I cannot emphasize strongly enough the need to obtain really pure essential oils if you are contemplating using them internally, such as for indigestion or heartburn.

PAIN RELIEF

Labour is so demanding and different from any other form of exercise that it is advisable to understand the processes involved and read some of the excellent childcare books currently available. Different groups of muscles will have a strenuous task during your labour, and the appropriate exercises which have been devised to strengthen these muscles should be regularly practised by anyone who wants to enjoy drug-free childbirth. One muscle which cannot be exercised in advance is the muscle of the cervix (the neck of the womb). It is this tight muscle which has to stretch open to allow the passage of the baby's head, and this is normally a slow and painful process; after all, it is that small but strong muscle which has held your baby inside the womb for the past nine months. Although I found that a back massage eased the general discomfort during contractions, I began to think that I couldn't handle the pain of the expanding cervix. It was when I was tempted to give in and ask for a general anaesthetic, that my husband applied a hand-hot **clary sage** compress to my lower abdomen, just above the pubic hair. Calendula tincture (a homoeopathic preparation) is equally effective. The relief from pain was instant and beyond my expectations, so that I neither wanted nor needed anything else for the duration of labour. As the compress cools down, it should be replaced with a fresh one, and obviously this can only be carried out while the woman is lying down. Some women prefer to move about during labour, and in that case a **clary sage** massage would be a good alternative to the compress (see page 153). Homoeopathic remedies can help to prepare your body for the process of childbirth, and I found that Caulophyllum strengthened and toned the womb, and with each of my children's births the pushing stage lasted only five minutes. For more information about homoeopathic remedies, see Bibliography.

Chapter Nine

AFTER THE BIRTH

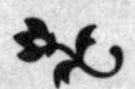

Because I have used essential oils as a matter of course after the birth of my three children, and have never experienced any post partum infection, I was very surprised to read a recent article in a nursing journal. The article was reporting on an epidemic of puerperal fever in a British maternity hospital, where several newly-delivered mothers had developed high fevers, having been infected with streptococcus. The cause of the infection was eventually traced to a hospital cleaner who was suffering from a chronic vaginal infection and had unwittingly charged the air with this infection. Antibiotics were given to all of the infected women, and I presume that the problem has been taken care of for the time being. However, if one member of staff can do so much damage, surely any visitor, nurse, doctor, or consultant, could do likewise, owing to the sad fact that staff often have to work while unwell, due to staff shortages. How many visitors would submit to a medical inspection every time they visited a person in hospital? Accepting that the atmosphere is never going to be sterile, but that mothers and babies are at risk and must be protected, should we not be insisting that essential oils be employed routinely in maternity hospitals? This could easily be done by giving the mothers regular sitz baths which incorporate essential oils, and by infusing essences into the atmosphere to combat airborne bacteria and viruses. Several British maternity hospitals encourage newly-delivered mothers to take aromatic baths, and the use of essential oils is acknowledged by midwives and nurses to be beneficial.

Another protective measure which I would like to see in the future, is for doctors, midwives and other staff directly in contact with newly-born babies, especially those babies who are premature and more vulnerable to infection, to gargle with antiseptic essential oils such as **lemon, bergamot** and **tea tree**, because the throat is usually the first site of infection.

After giving birth to my children, getting to know them and putting them to the breast, the first thing I did for myself was have a sitz bath with **cypress** and **lavender**. **Cypress** is astringent and causes the raw blood vessels to close over, and **lavender** oil is very healing, and gently encourages the growth of new skin at the same time as protecting the raw area from airborne infection. A new plastic bowl is ideal for a sitz bath. If you are small like me, then a washing up bowl if adequate. For larger ladies a baby bath would be necessary, or if it seems preferable, just two or three inches of water in a regular bath will suffice. Until the stitches were removed, I liked to have a sitz bath after every visit to the toilet. As the perineal skin heals more quickly when subjected to regular aromatic baths, the stitches (if any have been required) may thus disappear or (if necessary) be removed by the midwife a few days earlier.

Sore Nipples

Prevention is better than cure, and a regime for preparing the nipples for the onslaught of a hungry baby is definitely advisable. Babies have a very powerful grip, and suck extremely hard. I know of several women, who, although desperately keen to breast-feed their babies, were unable to because of the pain and the bleeding. Most of the essential oils are too strong for use on this sensitive area, and would also be inadvisable for the baby to swallow. In fact a nasty tasting oil may make the baby reject the breast. I would therefore recommend that only **lavender** or **rose** oil be used. A very dilute mix - one drop to one teaspoon nut oil - should be massaged into the nipples immediately after a feed and the nipples and aureola should be carefully washed before each feed.

After the Birth

Post-natal depression usually arrives with the milk, on day three or four after the birth. It is due to a hormone adjustment in the body, and most women get weepy and miserable for a day or two and then spontaneously recover; but a few unfortunate women suffer for months and months, to such a degree that they cannot feel any love for their child. My experience of post-natal depression was that of falling from a euphoric high into a bottomless pit of misery, from whose depths I was not able to see a way out. So intense was the experience that I was unable and unwilling to communicate and was totally unreasonable. Luckily for me, my husband knew that **jasmine** would be beneficial and ran a bath, to which he added a few drops of **jasmine**. I began to feel better almost as soon as I stepped into the bath and afterwards I went to sleep with a drop of **jasmine** oil on the edge of my pillow. When I woke up from my sleep, I was no longer suffering from post-natal depression, and was able to laugh at the way I had been just a few hours earlier.

If **jasmine** oil is not on hand, then **ylang-ylang** or **clary sage** oil are almost as effective.

Lactation Problems

Usually a woman's breasts produce milk spontaneously after the birth, and as the baby suckles, a further supply is generated: a case of supply and demand. Occasionally though, there is not enough milk to satisfy the baby's hunger. This could be due to an inadequate diet or depleted energies in the mother, possibly caused by a very exhausting labour, followed by nights of broken sleep, or maybe there are other children also demanding mother's attention. Fear of being unable to breast-feed can also impair the flow of milk.

Firstly the diet should be looked at to make sure that there are plenty of healthy and nutritious items, and that the total calorie intake is higher than for a non-breast-feeding woman. Your body can only produce milk from the raw materials you put into it.

Drinking a large glass of mineral water half an hour before the next feed is due, will help to ensure that the milk supply is adequate. The worst thing to do, if the milk supply is a little low, is to start supplementing the feed with a bottle of milk. This tends to produce the opposite effect to the desired one, either because the baby will demand less milk next time, and so less will be produced, or because baby has less effort to make to extract the milk from a bottle than from the breast, and may prefer a bottle.

On the few days when I experienced a lessened milk yield, I took **fennel** tea; easiest and cheapest way to buy an ounce or two of fennel seeds from a health food store and add a cup of water to 1 teaspoon fennel seed. Allow to stand for five minutes or so, strain and add a little honey if desired. Repeat every two hours. This will always work to increase the milk flow.

Mastitis

Sore breasts can be really painful and can even induce a high temperature. It used to be called 'milk fever' and was sometimes fatal. Mastitis is inflammation of the mammaries and can occur when the breast is not completely emptied of milk, or when a milk duct in the nipple gets clogged. It is a sensible idea to alternate which breast is offered to baby at the beginning of a feed, because the first breast given is always emptied, whereas the second one may not be, depending on the appetite of the baby. It is also important to wash the nipples carefully after every feed.

If mastitis should occur, then the most important thing is to reduce the heat in the local area. A compress of **lavender**, **geranium** and **rose** (see recipe on page 154) in tepid water will take away much of the heat and discomfort. If the temperature continues to rise, do consult a doctor. If symptoms of mastitis come on during the night and you decide to wait until morning before calling in the doctor, then the following can be employed. A **eucalyptus** footbath, together with the breast compress, will bring down the temperature temporarily, and this could be repeated every two hours. You should otherwise remain in bed, but do not allow yourself to get overheated with too many bedclothes. The breast compress should be freshly applied as necessary, and the nipple washed before feeding. If you feel strong enough, then have a **lavender** bath, with just comfortably warm water, but do get someone to help you in and out of the bath.

Mastitis also occurs when breast-feeding is stopped abruptly, as I found out one year. My second child was still asking for the breast when she was two years old, and it seemed possible that she would continue to breast-feed until she was school age. I went to stay with friends for a few days, leaving my husband to cope with the children. It was while I was away that my breasts became engorged, and I experienced all the classic symptoms of mastitis. By the time I arrived back home I was feeling really unwell, but by using the breast compresses and taking **lavender** baths I quickly returned to normal. Children adapt to changes much quicker than their mothers, and long before my temperature was back to 98.4, my daughter was happily drinking cups of soya milk.

TIREDNESS

Not being a marathon runner, or prima ballerina, and being totally unused to long hours of physical endurance, I have to say that labour was the most exhausting experience of my life. Labour is tiring for most women but with adequate rest and nutritious meals, the mother's strength should soon return. The time immediately after birth is one in which the mother needs help from other people. I had all of my babies at home, and was lucky to have a supportive husband and my own mother to offer me help. Although I desperately wanted to have my children at home, had I not had post partum help I would definitely have opted for a ten-day hospital stay. Immediately after childbirth is no time to start proving how tough you are. I say that from experience, having collapsed two weeks after the birth of my second child, and being 'put to bed' for almost a week. Such was my lack of vitality after my collapse, that it wasn't until after several weekly acupuncture treatments that I felt myself to be restored to my normal energy levels. After the birth, more than at any other time, is the time when a woman deserves a good massage. Labour is physically very demanding, and can take a lot out of you, but a back massage with a blend of essential oils (see recipe on page 154) will give renewed energy and strength, while removing much of the tension and strain caused to the back during the last months of pregnancy. A long labour, or an awkward birth, may also cause back pain which can persist for a long time, and any mother suffering in this way would be advised to visit a chiropractor.

Chapter Ten

Remedies for Children's Illnesses

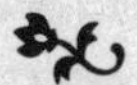

In this chapter I have used case histories from a variety of illnesses experienced by my own three children. Rarely have I called in the doctor, or taken the children to a surgery, but occasionally I have needed a second opinion. Often it is not necessary to wait until the illness develops to such a stage that a pathological change has occurred, making a diagnosis patently obvious. I find that it is far better to treat the child at the onset of an illness, either with homoeopathy, or with aromatherapy. My children are all teenagers and up until now not one of them has had a course of antibiotics, vaccinations or painkillers, and they have managed to survive a whole host of childhood ailments.

I am not suggesting that parents should abandon their doctors and treat all the serious diseases themselves, but I include this chapter for parents who, like me, believe that course after course of antibiotics, paracetamol and proprietory cough linctuses cannot be beneficial for their child, and prefer a more gentle and holistic treatment. I do recognize that antibiotics, those 'magic bullets' invented in the early twentieth century, have their uses. I was myself grateful for them on one occasion when a quinsy was closing my throat, and would welcome their use for my children should I ever encounter a problem which I cannot deal with.

Every ailment described in this chapter is one that I have encountered personally either in my own children or those of friends referred to me for advice. In my opinion, essential oils are perfectly capable of coping with a wide variety of health problems, and often they are all that is required, but I would like to point out that a knowledge of homoeopathy is a very valuable aid to any mother of young children. I always keep a wide selection of homoeopathic remedies, essential oils, and Bach Flower Remedies at home, and whenever I have to travel, I always take with me a small selection of the most important remedies.

Over the years, I have become quite expert at successfully treating myself and my family, and would not hesitate to treat any illness or health problem in my children or myself. However, I have a code of principles by which I work. The first has to be 'never take unnecessary risks': do call a doctor if an acute illness is not responding to your treatment and the life of your child is in jeopardy; be sensible, and take care of your own well-being, even while nursing a very sick child, by eating and resting; keep a cool head. If you are panicky and don't know what to do, then it is best to do nothing, and to seek the advice of a doctor.

You Are the Best Nurse

You are the best nurse that your child could ever have. You have the love that your child needs, and your presence is very important to a sick and frightened child. With all the best will in the world, a nurse cannot be a substitute for you, and love your child in the way you do. All you need is the confidence and knowledge to treat children's illnesses with the correct remedy, coupled with infinite amounts of patience.

My feeling is that children are vital, powerful beings, and when given the right help and support during an acute illness, their defence system will spring into action, and cope efficiently with the invading organism. I cannot see the necessity in prescribing antibiotics for little children every time they fall ill. When routinely given for acute illnesses which would respond just as quickly to gentler remedies, antibiotics become indiscriminate cell destroyers. Antibiotics disturb the natural balance of bowel flora, often killing the very bacillii vital to us if we are to have a healthy immune system. We are always going to be surrounded by viruses and germs of all descriptions, but as long as we have a strong immune system, we will be able to resist falling ill, or when we do become infected, will be able, with the help of aromatic oils, to shrug off the illness in a short period of time.

Dry Skin in Newborn Infants

When my son was born, his skin was somewhat dry and wrinkled, and he looked like a beautiful but tiny 'old man'. I did not want to use a mineral-based baby oil from a chemist (mineral oil is fine for rubbing on the buttocks, to guard against nappy rash, but not for treating dry skin) and instead chose to use **sweet almond** oil to which I added a little **rose** oil (see page 156).

A baby's skin is very delicate, and I do not advise the use of essential oils, except for a minute amount of **rose** and **lavender** oil in a base oil. This can be gently stroked into the parts of the body where the skin is dry. **Jojoba** is excellent at banishing dry skin, and has the added advantage, of leaving a very fine waxy coating, which will act as a barrier to moisture in the nappy area. Although I had not discovered the many benefits of **jojoba** when my children were babies, were I to have my family all over again, then **jojoba** would be an integral part of the nappy changing routine.

Colic

It is acceptable to be woken up three times a night to feed and change your baby, but something else altogether when they start screaming at about seven o'clock in the evening and continue well into the night. Nothing you do comforts the baby and the only recourse is to pace the floor until they drop off to sleep again. Three-month colic is not merely an old wives' tale. Once colic has established itself, it generally does not wear off until the infant is three months older; and that could be a lot of floor pacing.

Having found that a dose of proprietary gripe water did not cure the condition, but merely quietened the crying for up to one hour, I was not prepared for my new baby to be swallowing the quantities of sugar that gripe water contains, and decided to use a compress. **Camomile** was chosen for its soothing qualities, but it could just as easily have been **lavender** or **geranium**. Add one drop of essence to a small bottle of cold water and shake vigorously. Pour liquid into a glass bowl and top up with hot water until the temperature is comfortably warm. After mixing thoroughly, a handkerchief was wrung out in the **camomile** water, and applied to the baby's tummy. Then a small towel was placed on top of the compress to keep the area warm. After half an hour, or before that if the baby drops off to sleep, remove the compress. Take care to keep the baby warm.

Never be tempted to use more essential oil in the hope that it will work better or quicker. It will not. A baby's skin is very delicate, and this must always be respected.

Heat Bumps

Babies can easily get overheated during hot weather, and their way of letting mother know is to cry. Often the skin has little red bumps on it. Overheating can be dangerous if it leads to a convulsion, as this can sometimes result in brain damage. Heat bumps are nature's signal that something is wrong, and needs to be put right. The child should be undressed, and allowed to cool down. If it is convenient to bathe the child, then a lukewarm bath, to which one drop of **lavender** has been added, will be both cooling and calming.

Nosebleeds

When young children have a nosebleed, they usually become very frightened and sometimes even hysterical at the sight of their own blood. Adult remedies, such as putting a bunch of keys down the back, are not really suitable. **Lavender** would be the appropriate remedy. Put one or two drops of **lavender** into a small bowl of cold water, wring out a handkerchief in the liquid, and lay it over the bridge of the nose. The bleeding should stop very quickly and, because of the soothing properties of **lavender**, the child will soon be calmed. The first-aid treatment, if you were out in the car, would be to place a drop of **lavender** oil on the corner of a tissue, and insert it gently into the affected nostril.

TOOTHACHE

If children are not given too many sweets and fizzy drinks, then the likelihood of toothache is remote, but there may be an occasion when a tooth aches, and perhaps there is a day or so to wait before a visit to a dentist can be arranged. For the older child, a drop of **clove** or **peppermint** oil on a small piece of cotton wool, and placed on the affected tooth, will take away some of the pain. I have also found that when **clove** oil is rubbed into the gum, it anaesthetizes the pain. Because of the strong taste, it would not be suitable for a very young child, and in this instance a **lavender** compress would be more acceptable. Put one drop of **lavender** in warm water, then apply the moist cloth to the face, over the sore spot, and keep the area warm.

Teething babies will stop crying and go to sleep when a drop of **lavender** or **camomile** oil is placed on the edge of their pillow. Also putting a drop on the front of the nightie or pyjamas - so that the vapours can be inhaled - will calm down a fractious child.

Note: When an oil is placed on a baby's pillow or clothing, care must be taken to ensure that the oil does not come into direct contact with the baby's skin.

EARACHE

Earache was a particularly distressing part of my childhood. I seemed to have recurrent bouts of it, and was given salt packs, cotton wool soaked in castor oil, and aspirin. None of these seemed to work very well, and I wish that my mother had known about **lavender**. One drop on a small piece of cotton wool and placed gently in the outer ear, will work wonders. The healing vapours find their way into the inner ear and take away the pain. Earache may be caused by a subluxation of the bones of the neck or an energy block, in which case a permanent cure will only be effected by acupuncture, chiropractic or manipulation. (See Useful Addresses at the end of the book.)

COLDS AND FLU

At the first signs of 'stuffiness' in my children, I would put them to bed with a drop of **eucalyptus** oil on the outer edges of the pillow. Sometimes this treatment alone is sufficient to stop the cold from progressing. **Eucalyptus** has the ability to unblock the stuffiest of noses, but do have lots of tissues handy!

For influenza-type colds, the **eucalyptus** treatment will not suffice. In 1989, the year of the flu epidemic, my children reported that classes of 30-plus in their schools were reduced to ten pupils. Each of my children became ill with the flu, and to alleviate the sore neck and aching backs, I rubbed in a little neat **lavender** oil. I also massaged their chests with **lavender** oil, paying particular attention to the space between the ribs. I have found that pain is only experienced when there is an infection, and that by gently massaging the sore spots, the child soon begins to feel better, and has more energy. There are many lymph nodes across the chest, and soreness in these areas denotes that they are fighting the infection. A little **lavender** will give assistance to that part of the body which needs it most.

My youngest child had a very constricted throat, and became quite panicky in the middle of one night. I rubbed lots of **lavender** into the lymph nodes in the neck and under the jaw, and also used acupressure/shiatsu holding techniques. (These hurt at first, but as the pain subsided, the underlying ache had been lessened.) Rubbing a little **lavender** oil into the nape of the neck will do much to relieve the headache which accompanies flu.

I was determined not to succumb to the virus, even though I could feel its presence in my neck and throat, and did to myself what I have already described above. I carried on with work as normal, without the need for a day in bed. During the ten days it took for my family to recovery fully, I kept hearing reports of the hundreds of fatalities attributed to the flu epidemic, and I was saddened and angered at such wastage of life. It surely begs the question, 'Is it not time for the medical establishment to test the validity of the therapeutic claims made for essential oils?'

Note: The holding technique Ning entails pinching the flesh between the second segments of the first and second fingers. Practise doing it on your own neck, so that you have experienced the benefit of putting up with a little pain, and can convince your child that you know what you are doing (see Bibliography, *Quick and Easy Chinese Massage*).

INFECTED SINUSES

The sinuses are an important part of our voice resonance, and when infected, as they usually are during a common cold, the voice sounds quite dull and flat, and we say that we have a 'stuffy nose'. Usually when the cold has cleared up, the sinus cavities, in the bones surrounding the nose, return to normal. Sometimes the sinuses are infected for extended periods of time, causing headaches, earache or 'faceache', and making the sufferer feel uncomfortable and irritable.

Allergies such as hay fever, intolerance of house dust, and even food allergies can cause sinusitis. My son, who is allergic to dairy products, and sensitive to cigarette smoke and traffic fumes, often has infected sinuses. I have found that **lavender** oil, gently massaged into the sinuses at either side of the nose, will clear up the condition in a few days. Even more spectacular results, though, are obtained by using a little-known oil called **inula**. Inula must be well diluted in **jojoba** or a nut oil (see recipe section), but when gently rubbed into the sinuses, the infection is cleared up within 24 hours. I have found that only two or three applications are necessary.

Inula is wonderful for curing sinusitis, whether acute or chronic, and as changes in altitude can make infected sinuses feel very uncomfortable, I would recommend it to all air travellers, and especially to airline staff.

CONJUNCTIVITIS

When eyes become inflamed, exuding a sticky discharge, and the white turns pink, the condition is known as conjunctivitis. Several years ago, when my children were younger and had a rabbit called Bunnykins, one of the children and the rabbit had conjunctivitis at the same time. I never did find out who infected whom, but treated them both with aromatherapy. I used pure **lavender** oil in water (diluting 2-3 drops of **lavender** in a 500ml bottle of lukewarm water and shaking it vigorously) and with cotton wool balls, gently bathed the eye, stroking downwards from the top of the eyelid, across the lashes, and onto the cheekbone. Several new pieces of cotton wool may be needed before the eye has been cleansed, and strict attention should be placed on hygiene and the used cotton wool placed in a plastic bag, to avoid cross-infection. **Lavender** is very gentle, and neither my child nor the rabbit made any fuss. I needed to bathe my child's eyes three times before the condition was cleared, but the rabbit was able to open his eyes after the first treatment, and after the second treatment was completely cured.

TETCHINESS AND TANTRUMS

If children do not have a sound night's sleep, for whatever reason, after a bad dream, a wet bed, or feeling sick during the night, they can be pretty hard to handle the following morning. Many years ago when my children were small and one of them had woken up in a 'don't want to eat breakfast/get dressed/go to school' mood, I found that the simplest thing to do was run a shallow bath, add a drop or two of **clary sage** oil, and leave the child there for ten minutes. The difference in attitude was incredible. Each time I used this remedy for a grumpy child, there was a transformation, with the moodiness turning into smiles before the child had left the bathroom. **Clary sage** is a hormonal regulator, and if disturbed sleep produces a hormone which triggers depression, this could explain why **clary sage** has such a wonderful effect. **Clary sage** has been known as a euphoric for many years.

FEVER

When fever occurs, it is nature's way of fighting infection, and therefore should not be suppressed. However, sometimes the fever prevents the child from getting to sleep, and then it is prudent to alleviate the discomfort by giving the child a lukewarm bath, to which 3 to 4 drops of **lavender** have been added. On the occasions when I have used this treatment, the **lavender** bath soothes, cools and calms the child, allowing him or her to feel comfortable and relaxed, and therefore able to fall asleep easily.

If a child's temperature reaches very high levels (103°F/39°C) or more and you cannot bring down the temperature, then a doctor should be consulted. But I have found that even seriously high temperatures can be reduced and controlled with the use of certain essential oils. Once when my son, then one year old, had a high temperature, I wrapped his feet in **eucalyptus** compresses (two drops of **eucalyptus** in a bowl of cold water), and renewed with fresh ones as the compresses became warm. In this way I was able to nurse him back from a dangerously high fever to a safe level in a very short space of time, and without the need for medical assistance. There is always a danger that a child may start convulsing if the body temperature goes too high, and actively to work towards normalizing the body heat is much less stressful to parents, than to sit by the bedside watching helplessly as the temperature climbs higher and higher.

CHICKEN POX

To help a child throw off the chicken pox virus, I would not hesitate to recommend that he or she be given a homoeopathic remedy just as soon as the virus has manifested itself on the skin. My first choice would be homoeopathic Rhus Tox. Prompt treatment can, and does, clear up chicken pox in under one week. However, there is still the problem of itching, and it is difficult to prevent a child from scratching. This can lead to permanent damage to the skin, in the form of the little dents, known commonly as 'pock marks'. As each of my children went down with chicken pox (thankfully not simultaneously), I dosed them with the homoeopathic remedy, and dabbed their skin with an essential oil lotion. Knowing that **peppermint** oil was cooling and soothing, but not wishing to put my spotty youngsters into a bath, I made up a lotion to apply to the skin: to 1 litre bottle of water I added 1 drop of **peppermint** oil, and then shook the bottle vigorously. I then tipped out half the contents, topped up with water and shook the bottle again. I then repeated the procedure, so that I ended up with ¼ drop of **peppermint** oil in 1 litre of water. (I could just as easily have used **lavender** oil.) By diluting and shaking the lotion, I was actually following the basic homoeopathic principles of attenuation, and possibly I achieved a low-potency homoeopathic remedy. However, my concern was to make a very dilute peppermint wash, as I am quite aware of the homoeopathic precept which states that **peppermint** will antidote all homoeopathic remedies. Following my intuition however, I duly applied the very weak solution to the spots, using cotton wool. My son, who had been very fidgety and itchy, immediately noticed the difference, and did not feel the need to scratch any more. Having been successful with my first 'guinea pig', I subsequently used the same lotion on my two daughters when they developed chicken pox, with equally good results.

Lavender has been used equally successfully, by a relative of mine, who contracted chicken pox while staying with friends. She was a young teenager and was very worried that she might scratch herself and become scarred. She only had **lavender** oil with her, and knowing that **lavender** has many uses, applied it in the same way that I had used **peppermint**. The chicken pox cleared up in the normal time span, and she was pleased that the itching had been soothed, and that no scratching had been necessary.

Note: I have spoken with prominent homoeopaths about the possible negating effect of essences on homoeopathic remedies, and so far, there does not seem to be a standard opinion.

Whooping Cough

Respiratory diseases can be very frightening to both the child and the parents, because of the constriction of the airways. Whooping cough is caused by a bacteria, and the allopathic remedy given is usually a course of anti-biotics. However, when my child went down with whooping cough, my GP was aware of my antipathy towards anti-biotics and recommended 'good nursing' as my course of action. The outcome of an acute disease such as whooping cough depends on whether or not a child has a strong constitution. Homeopathy is one therapy which can augment and strengthen the immune system, thereby helping the child to fight the infection and recovery quickly. I used steam vapours in the sick room, to which I had added some essential oils. Any one of the anti-spasmodic essential oils would do - **basil**, **clary sage**, **cypress**, **eucalyptus**, **juniper**, **lavender** or **rosemary**. One or two drops in a bowl of hot water will be beneficial to the sick child. I also used a warm **lavender** compress on the chest, to aid the body's fight against the virus and also to relax and soothe a terrified little girl.

The chest compress should be made by using warm water to which 1 or 2 drops of **lavender** have been mixed. A handkerchief or face flannel is then dipped into the water, wrung, and placed on the chest. To keep the child comfortably warm, a dry fluffy towel should be placed over the compress, and when cool should be removed or replaced with a fresh, warm compress. By taking an active role in the treatment of your sick child, there is less opportunity for you, the parent, to become distressed, and a calm mother will help ensure that the child remains calm, which is most important when treating spasmodic disorders.

Note: whooping cough is highly infectious and there should be no contact with other children, in order to minimize the spread of the disease.

Before my children were born, their father and I made a decision to bring up our children without vaccination or immunization, after having read a book called *The Blood Poisoners*. Even though two of my children suffered an acute attack of whooping cough, I have never regretted our decision.

There are other reasons to avoid the vaccination programme (see Bibliography).

Infantile Eczema

Hydro-cortisone is regularly prescribed for skin conditions ranging from nappy rash to chronic eczema. It permanently changes the skin texture if used over long periods, making the skin leathery. It does not cure eczema, but suppresses the disease, driving it inwards.

Often eczema is linked to asthma and I was afraid of this when my son (now an adult) was a baby. He had been breast-fed and was a perfect baby to look at until the age of six months, when I introduced him to a baby cereal containing dried milk powder - our troubles began. Along with the eczema, James had diarrhoea, lost weight, and was admitted to hospital, where he had to undergo many tests, until the doctors had satisfied themselves that he was intolerant of cow's milk. When given a brand of soya bean milk, he began to recover, and put on weight, but the eczema remained. The eczema was so bad that it covered almost all of his body and face, and was so irritating for James that he scratched his face until it bled, and I had to put a square of muslin between his face and my clothing before I could cuddle him.

James was diagnosed as having very severe eczema, and I was given hydro-cortisone cream, which I declined to use, even though it meant that I was criticized in the strongest terms, by the hospital doctors. Having great faith in homoeopathy, but not in my knowledge of the subject, I took James to the homoeopathic hospital in Great Ormond Street, where he was treated as an outpatient for almost a year. Externally, I soothed his skin with Calendula cream and Dr Bach's Rescue Remedy Cream, and with **lavender** baths (only 1 or 2 drops of **lavender** oil to an average bath). His eczema did not clear up overnight, but by the time James started school, his skin complaint was confined to his hands, behind his knees, a little on his back, and patches around his mouth. By the age of 11 years, and entering senior school, the problem had been reduced to occasional itching of the fingers, and by the age of 16 years, he was free of eczema, although mild symptoms return if ever he is tempted to eat milk chocolate or ice cream.

With love and patience, together with gentle remedies, even the most distressing of skin complaints can be cured. I mean *really* cured, not just suppressed. You need to be strong, to sometimes take a stand against the medical persuasiveness to use drugs, and to have faith in the unlauded, often unseen, and softly spoken remedies of nature.

Asthma

Asthma in children is something I have never had dealings with, although I was told by doctors that my son with eczema would inevitably develop asthma.

Very often I have heard of asthmatic children being allergic to specific items of food, and now that the medical profession recognizes that food allergies do exist, and do pose health problems, it is worth finding out which foods (or other substances) are causing the problem.

Many of the essential oils are anti-spasmodic and soothing to the respiratory tract, and once I found that the blend of essences given to my accountant to make his office environment more pleasant was beneficial in preventing a colleague of his from having an asthmatic attack. (See recipe on page 156). However it sometimes happens that essential oil vapours can aggravate an asthmatic attack. Do consult a qualified practitioner before treating an asthmatic child.

Aching Legs

When your child wakes up in the middle of the night, crying and moaning about 'achy legs' it is no comfort to the child or to you, to be told that it is 'just growing pains'. It is normally the calf muscles which are sore, or in spasm, but I do not know why it happens to some children and not others. Two of my three children have been affected in this way, and the entire household has been woken by the distressed youngster. I usually give the child a homoeopathic remedy such as Arnica, and also massage the leg with an essential oil blend, which I keep for such emergencies. This treatment has always worked well. (See recipe on page 155.)

Stomach Ache

It is not often now that my children have tummy aches, but they tended to be the norm after having attended birthday parties when they were younger. Everything that is sweet and gooey and normally rationed, is suddenly available in vast quantities, and what child can resist? It was normally on getting into bed, that the moaning and groaning would start, followed by cries of 'I feel sick'.

My remedy for tummy aches is always the same. I dissolve a teaspoon of honey into ½ cup of warm water, and then add one drop of **peppermint** oil, and stir again. As it is too strong, even for me, to drink from the cup, I spoon it into my child. **Peppermint** vapours are very powerful, and my youngest child always had to take a deep breath first, close her eyes and then swallow the **peppermint** water. However, just a few teaspoonsfuls of the mixture will settle the stomach.

Convulsions

A doctor should always be called if a child goes into convulsions, but while you are waiting for your doctor to arrive there are certain things you can do. Remove all the child's clothing and place him or her into a lukewarm **lavender** bath, supporting the head with one hand and gently wetting the child's body with the water. Just a few minutes is long enough, and then wrap the child in a large bath towel, to prevent chilling. As a convulsing child is a frightening sight, I recommend that the parents should take a dose of Rescue Remedy to allay their panic.

When the young daughter of a friend of mine went into convulsion, Lizzie carried out the treatment as above, and by the time the doctor arrived the child was sitting up and smiling. Lizzie wasn't sure whether she should be apologizing to the doctor for wasting his time, or thankful to the **lavender** for working so promptly.

HEADACHE (SEVERE)

Children do not get very severe headaches unless they are extremely ill, or have sunstroke or concussion from a fall. It is therefore wise to telephone a doctor and describe the symptoms. Never administer an adult painkiller.

One night in 1983 my youngest daughter, then aged four, woke up crying about a sore head. The next 48 hours had all the ingredients of every parent's worst nightmare. I still do not know for certain whether Saffron had meningitis, but I shall describe the circumstances surrounding the illness.

First thing in the morning I rang the nursery school to say that Saffron would not be in, and was told that the Principal of the school had meningitis, and was in the intensive care unit of the local hospital. During the day Saffron's temperature increased, she was prostrate, crying continually and vomiting each time I gave her a drink. I noticed that she was photophobic (had an inversion to light), had a very sore back, and could not bend her neck. Whether by good luck or bad luck, this illness occurred within a few months of us moving from Oxford to Brighton, and I had not registered with a local doctor. My immediate choices seemed to be either to call an ambulance or to treat the condition myself, while going through the formalities of registering with a doctor. I called a homoeopathic doctor friend of mine, who recommended a high potency of homoeopathic Pulsatilla, and to get Saffron assessed by a doctor as soon as possible. The Pulsatilla was fast-acting and by the end of the day, all of the symptoms had lessened in severity, except the headache which prevented Saffron from sleeping. I decided to use a **lavender** compress across the forehead, as

lavender is sedative, but it did not produce the desired effect. I then thought of using **geranium**, as it is neither sedative nor stimulating, but has a harmonizing action. I was stunned. The instant I laid the **geranium** soaked cloth across the forehead, Saffron murmured, 'Oh, mummy, that smells nice' and dropped off to sleep. She slept for the remainder of that day, and was able to drink small amounts of pure water, and had quite a good night's sleep. Our new doctor arrived the following morning, but as Saffron was no longer photophobic, and could bend her neck slightly, she was diagnosed as having a virus which displayed similar symptoms to meningitis, but which was not meningitis! I was overjoyed to hear that diagnosis, because it meant that homoeopathy and aromatherapy had averted the almost certain need for hospitalization and lumbar punctures. I don't mind admitting that I was hardly dry-eyed for two days, and would never want to re-live that experience, but at the same time, I am thankful that I have witnessed the power of these natural remedies in a critical situation.

HEAD LICE

If you have children at playgroup or school, you will undoubtedly have encountered the dreaded head lice. When my children were infected (and one-for-all, all-for-one seems to be the head lice motto) I decided to try a treatment with essential oils (see page 155).

I sectioned the hair from the forehead to the neck, and applied the 'lice mixture' to the scalp, until the entire head had been covered in this way, making sure that all of the hair had been covered. I then piled the hair on top of the head and wrapped a long sheet of clingfilm tightly around the head, and behind the ears. I was not sure how my children would endure this treatment but they loved it, and scampered about the house being 'space-invaders' for a couple of hours! When the clingfilm was removed over the bath, most of the 'problem' went with it. The next step was a good hair-wash. As with all oily hair treatments, shampoo needs to be applied first, to make an emulsion, and then water added. After thoroughly washing the hair I used the regulation fine-toothed 'nit comb', to dislodge any eggs which might have adhered to the hair strands. I repeated this treatment after three days, and again after a further five days, to ensure that I caught anything which might have subsequently hatched. (Lice eggs are not only stuck to the hair shaft with super-glue, but they are impervious to any preparation, and don't become vulnerable until they have hatched.) A welcome side-effect of the lice treatment was that my children were the owners of lustrous, shining, healthy hair.

PRE-PARTY NERVES

Adults are not the only ones to suffer from pre-party nerves and, with children, the eagerly anticipated party suddenly produces floods of tears and pleas to stay at home. If either of my daughters became upset prior to a party, I would pop her into a **geranium** bath (two drops), as it always relaxed them and took away the anxiety.

Just as perfume gives a boost to our morale, so can a perfume help young children to overcome their nervousness and help them to cope with new situations. A blend of essential oils suitable for use as a perfume can easily be concocted in a few minutes. Dilution of the essential oils is a 'must' before use, and as I did not wish to use an alcohol base for a child's perfume, I chose **jojoba** oil. **Jojoba**, being a liquid wax, does not oxidize, and therefore the unused perfume will last for a very long time. (See page 156.)

SORE THROATS

The throat is the first site of infection for most airborne bacteria and viruses, and many diseases begin life as a simple sore throat. **Tea tree** oil has antiseptic properties, while being non-damaging to skin tissue, and is therefore an ideal first-aid treatment. Whenever one of my children has a sore throat, I get them to gargle with **tea tree**. To a glass of water (two-thirds full), add one drop of **tea tree** oil, cover the top of the glass with your hand or a clean cloth, and shake vigorously. Very young children have difficulty in grasping the techniques of gargling, without spluttering and swallowing some of the mixture. **Tea tree** is safe for internal use, and therefore if any is swallowed no harm will occur.

Children, and indeed adults who have had their tonsils removed, have lost an important part of the total defence system of the body. The tonsils do not actually produce the cells which fight infection. These cells are produced in the thymus and the bone marrow, which are known as Primary Lymphatic Organs. The cells then travel to other parts of the body such as the spleen and tonsils (the Secondary Lymphatic Organs), where they are given specific tasks; i.e. to become B cells which produce antibodies or to become T-helper, T-suppressor, or natural killer cells (NK). Each of these cells have their specific jobs to do, but they also interrelate to work as a whole, in protecting us from disease. When we have lost an important part of this system, such as the tonsils or appendix, it becomes even more necessary to help our body to function efficiently when under attack, by using those essential oils which destroy bacteria and fungi and which can work with and aid our defence systems in fighting infection.

Niaouli is an excellent oil for fighting throat infections, as well as relieving a ticklish cough. The simplest way of administering **niaouli** is as a **niaouli** cough mixture - see page 155.

WARTS AND VERRUCAS

Children seem to be more susceptible than adults to catching warts and verrucas, probably because - as part of the education system - they are barefoot two or three times a week as they undergo physical education, swimming lessons, or just walking around the changing room after football or netball.

Once many years ago my youngest child showed me a wart on one of her feet. It was right on the tip of a little toe, as though it had been stuck on with glue. Each evening, before bedtime, I applied a little neat **lemon** oil. I dripped **lemon** oil onto the very corner of a tissue, and then gently touched the tissue to the centre of the wart. There were a few squeals of discomfort, but we persevered for a little more than a week. On about the eighth or ninth day of treatment, I went to apply the **lemon** but there was no wart, nor any sign of where the wart had been. Whereupon my daughter quite nonchalantly said: 'Oh mummy, I forgot to tell you, it just dropped off.'

Verrucas are more tricky to get rid of, and care should be taken that the verruca is covered over with a clean plaster each day, to avoid spreading the problem to other members of the family. Oils to treat a verruca could either be **tea tree, lemon** or **lavender.** The skin surrounding the verruca should not be allowed to become hard and dry, but should be bathed daily, and any dead material in the centre of the verruca should be removed carefully. Then a little oil should be rubbed into the verruca, and covered with a sticking plaster to which a drop of oil has been added.

Note: normally I would not use **lemon** oil for children, as, with the other citrus oils, it can be a little irritating to the skin. However, it is, in my opinion, unsurpassed when used for curing warts.

Chapter Eleven

BLENDING

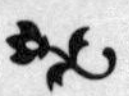

If we are using two or more essences in a blend, it is important to choose correctly, in order to prepare a harmonious blend. There are certain essences which 'marry' perfectly, thus improving the overall effect. Conversely, some essences do not blend well together, and then we have an unharmonious aroma. The correct choice of essence, and the blending together of those essences to enhance the powers of the oils, is called synergy.

From the information in the various aromatherapy books, it is fairly easy to pinpoint which oils are recommended for a particular problem. However, out of that list of therapeutic oils, there will be some which do not blend well together, and some which do. So, how do we find the synergistic blend?

The way in which I find the correct blend of essences is as follows.

First I take some strips of blotting paper (about ½cm/¼in wide by 12cm/5in long), one for each of the oils which I have shortlisted. Then I put a drop of essence on to one of the paper strips, and write the name of the essence at the opposite end of the strip. I continue to do this until I have one strip of paper impregnated with an essence, for every essence which I am considering. I decide which is the most important essence (for example, **lavender**) and call this the 'key' essence. Next to this I place one of the other strips, so that they are close, but not touching (see diagram on page 137). I then smell the two together and decide whether the aromas harmonize with each other. If this second essence does not smell right with my 'key', then I discard the second essence and hold number three next to the 'key'. Thus I continue to add further essences to the collection in my hand, discarding those which do

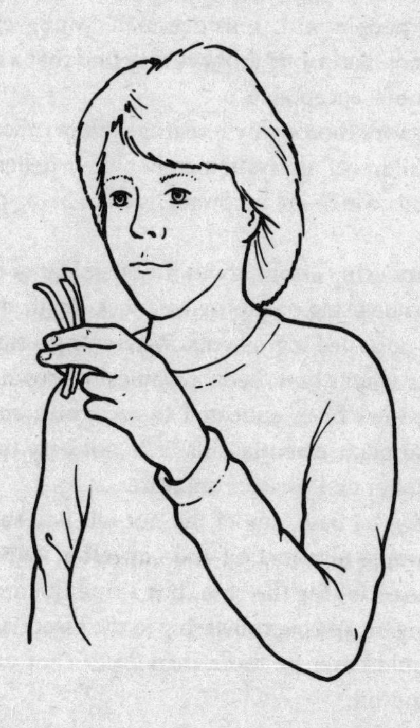

not harmonize, until I have tried all of the strips, and I am satisfied with the harmony of the blend. Then I will work out in what proportion I want the essential oils to be blended, and then mix them together. If the finished 'perfume' is right, then whether the resulting blend is for the bath, a massage oil, a facial oil, an inhalation or perfume, the person who uses it will respond in a positive way. If you have all of the right therapeutic ingredients, but the finished product does not smell pleasing, then the recipient will unconsciously reject the treatment. If it is not *pleasant* then it is *unpleasant.*

When using essential oils, please always remember that they are powerful and concentrated and just because a little is beneficial, it does not mean that a large amount will work better. Only tiny amounts should be used.

A 2 per cent dilution of essential oils is the maximum that should be used. Many people with sensitive skin, young children, and people who do not like strong aromas, may find that a more diluted blend will be more acceptable.

Some oils are more thoroughly researched than others, and when using oils for children I always remember their delicate skin, and only use those oils which are recommended as being gentle on the skin.

Whether we are using essential oils for ourselves or our children, it is important to be using only pure essences, distilled from plants, and which have no added ingredients. Wherever possible, try to buy oils from plants which have been organically grown.

Once the nose has been educated to recognize and appreciate the smell of real plant essential oils, it is not easy to fool it with synthetic or adulterated essence mixtures.

For the massage oil base, any of the nut oils will suffice, but my favourites are **sweet almond** oil and **camellia. Olive** oil may be used and is wonderful for the skin, but I find the aroma of **olive** oil to be too pungent and overpowering to the essential oils. A facial massage oil should never be more than 2 per cent essential oil to 98 per cent base oil.

Dos and Don'ts of Blending

Wash hands before and after blending essential oils. Always remember that essential oils are concentrated, and are not intended to be used neat on the skin, so wash off any spills.

Replace the caps on the bottles as soon as you have counted out the drops. This will ensure that: (a) the caps of different bottles do not get mixed up, and (b) that the essential oils do not evaporate into the atmosphere.

Count the drops as they are added to the bottle, keeping a record on a piece of paper. It is easy to lose concentration - maybe the phone will ring - and you may not remember whether or not you have added such and such an oil.

Add the **jojoba** and nut/seed oil to the essential oil blend.

Remember that essential oil blends are badly affected by heat, light, oxygen, and moisture. So keep them in dark bottles, well stoppered, and out of direct sunlight.

The massage oil base may be made from any nut or seed oil, such as **safflower**; **sunflower**; **sweet almond**; **peach kernel**; **grape seed** oil. **Olive** oil may be used, but I find that the aroma is overpowering to the essential oils.

Aromatic Water

An essence in water can be used for the following:

- Facial cleanser/toner
- Compress - tummy ache; foot compress to reduce fever; face compress (after a facial massage).
- Freshener during hot weather; hand wash (keep in the car for emergencies, such as spilt petrol on the hands; mopping up after a sick child; etc).

Face cleanser/compress: 1-3 drops of essential oil in 100ml water (preferably bottled).

Freshener/hand wash: 5-6 drops of essential oil in 100ml water.

Add the drops of essential oil to a bottle of water, and shake well. As the essence will not dissolve, but only disperse, it will be necessary to shake the bottle before each use.

Chapter Twelve

RECIPES

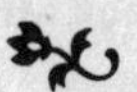

DECIDING ON QUANTITY

Whether to make up a small bottle of massage oil or instead to just make enough for one massage will depend largely upon what ailment is being treated. For example, a massage oil to treat period pains is only going to be used once a month and therefore it would be preferable to just make enough for one application. Conversely, if treating skin which is covered with acne, a daily application of massage oil will be needed for a considerable length of time. In the latter case it would be preferable to make up between 30 and 100ml. Some useful conversions are given on page 163.

Throughout the recipe chapter I have given recipes for a bottle of massage oil as well as for a single application.

Recipes for Chapter One

Muscular aches

(massage oil)

10 drops **juniper**
7 drops **lavender**
8 drops **rosemary**
in 50ml base oil

or

2 drops **juniper**
1 drop **lavender**
1 drop **rosemary**
in 2 teaspoons base oil

Hangover

(bath)

2 drops **juniper**
1 drop **rosemary**

Bergamot tea (Earl Grey)
1 teaspoon of black tea
1 drop of **bergamot**
3-4 cups of hot water

Lemon tea
1 teaspoon of black or green tea
1 drop of **lemon**
1-2 cups of hot water

Aromatic teas

Peppermint tea
1 teaspoon of black tea
1 drop of **peppermint**
3-4 cups of hot water

Orange tea
1 teaspoon of black or green tea
1 drop of **orange**
1-2 cups of hot water

Recipes for Chapter Two

Period pains
(massage oil)
15-20 drops **clary sage**
in 50ml base oil

or

2 drops **clary sage** oil
1 teaspoon fatty oil
Massage into the lower abdomen, lower back and groin area.

Leucorrhoea
(douche)
As for thrush.

Cystitis
(lotion)
1 drop **lavender**
in 100ml water. Make up a small plastic bottle, and shake well before each use.

Herpes
(massage oil)
for applying to the glands at the top inside leg
1 drop **rose**
2 drops **lavender**
in 2 teaspoons base oil
(or **jojoba**)

Pruritus
(sitz bath)
1 drop **rose**
1 drop **peppermint**
in bowl of warm water (large enough to sit in)

Thrush

(douche)

2 drops **rose**
4 drops **lavender**
2 drops **bergamot**
in 1 litre warm water. Shake well in a bottle. Add to douche/enema pot.

Thrush

(douche)

6 drops **tea tree**
in 1 litre warm water. Shake well in a bottle. Add to douche/enema pot.

Vaginal pessary

1 small tampon
several drops of **tea tree**
Remove tampon from its wrapper, and drop **tea tree** oil across the top and sides (down about 1cm). Insert as you would during menstruation. These pessaries should be changed at least twice in 24 hours, and will clear up many minor vaginal problems within a day or two. *Lavender* oil may be substituted for **tea tree** oil. It is recommended that only one pessary at a time be made up, ensuring sterility of tampon, and also that the **tea tree** oil does not evaporate.

Recipes for Chapter Three

Thigh slimmer

(massage oil)

10 drops **cypress**
10 drops **juniper**
5 drops **lavender**
in 50ml base oil
(the addition of some **jojoba** is very beneficial)

or

1 drop **cypress**
1 drop **juniper**
1 drop **lavender**
in 10ml base oil
(preferably at least 50 per cent **jojoba**)

Breast developer

(massage oil)

9 drops **geranium**
16 drops **ylang-ylang**
in 50ml base oil
(do not use **jojoba)**

or

2 drops **geranium**
1 drop **ylang-ylang**
in 2 teaspoon **camellia**
(or other base oil)

Aphrodisiac massage oil

5 drops **jasmine**
5 drops **rose**
10 drops **sandalwood**
5 drops **bergamot**
in 50ml base oil

or

1 drop **jasmine**
1 drop **rose**
2 drops **sandalwood**
1 drop **bergamot**
in 2 teaspoons base oil

or

1 drop **ylang-ylang**
1 drop **sandalwood**
1 drop **myrtle**
in 2 teaspoons **camellia** base

or

1 drop **clary sage**
1 drop **sandalwood**
1 drop **myrtle**
in 2 teaspoons **camellia** base

A heady, jasmine perfume

2 drops **jasmine**
12 drops **rosewood**
6 drops **ylang-ylang**
in 10ml **jojoba**
(see 'Rose perfume')

Eau de Cologne

20 drops **petitgrain** or **neroli**
80 drops **bergamot**
30 drops **lemon**
40 drops **orange**
20 drops **lavender**
10 drops **rosemary**

Add to distilled water, or better still use pure spring bottled water.

For a stronger scent, add the essential oils to 100ml of water.

For a more subtle aroma, add the essential oils to 200ml of water.

The mixture should be taken before each use.

A rose perfume

4 drops **rose**
12 drops **sandalwood**
2 drops **geranium**
2 drops **rosewood**
in 10ml **jojoba** (This is too strong to be used for massage, and should be applied sparingly as you would a perfume.)

Jasmine tea

1 teaspoon of green tea
1 drop **jasmine**
3-4 cups of hot water
Serve immediately.
(Ensure that the **jasmine** is pure. Pure **jasmine** is expensive but well worth tracking down. A small bottle can last for many years.)

Bedroom to boudoir

Lashings of exotic essences to perfume the atmosphere - (**jasmine, rose, patchouli, sandalwood, ylang-ylang, myrtle, clary sage**)
Just add imagination.

Recipes for Chapter Five

Resistance builder

(massage oil)
20 drops **lavender**
5 drops **bergamot**
in 50ml base oil

or

2 drops **lavender**
1 drop **bergamot**
2 teaspoons base oil

or

7 drops **tea tree**
7 drops **lavender**
7 drops **bergamot**
4 drops **sandalwood**
in 50ml base oil

or

1 drop **tea tree**
1 drop **lavender**
1 drop **sandalwood**
1 drop **bergamot**
in 2 teaspoons base oil

Mouthwash

1 drop **peppermint**
1 drop **lemon**
in 200ml water
(Shake well in a bottle. If pure water is used, and the bottle is tightly capped, the mixture will last for several weeks.)

Relaxing massage oil

13 drops **lavender**
2 drops **geranium**
10 drops **sandalwood**
in 50ml base oil
or
2 drops **lavender**
1 drop **geranium**
2 drops **sandalwood**
in 2 teaspoons base oil
or for an even more sedative formula
10 drops **geranium**
10 drops **lavender**
5 drops **marjoram**
in 50ml base oil
or
1 drop **geranium**
2 drops **lavender**
2 drops **marjoram**
in 2 teaspoons base oil

Invigorating massage oil

17 drops **rosewood**
6 drops **orange**
2 drops **geranium**
in 50ml base oil
or
3 drops **rosewood**
2 drops **orange**
1 drop **geranium**
in 2 teaspoons base oil
or
12 drops **rosemary**
9 drops **clary sage**
4 drops **myrtle**
in 50ml base oil

Shingles

(**peppermint/lavender** lotion)
1 drop **peppermint** or **lavender**
1 litre bottle of water
Add peppermint to water, cap and shake vigorously. Pour away half of the contents. Refill with water. Cap and shake. Pour away half the contents. Refill with water. You are now left with ¼ drop of **peppermint** oil to 1 litre of water. This is cooling to hot, itchy skin, and because the dilution is so weak, it should not antidote any homoeopathic remedies being taken.

Geranium oil may be used in place of **peppermint** or **lavender**.

Depression

(pick-me-up bath)
2 drops **clary sage**
2 drops **bergamot**
2 drops **ylang-ylang**
Add to bath water, mix well.

Glandular tonic

(massage oil)
5 drops **tea tree**
5 drops **lavender**
in 10ml **jojoba**
(or other base oil if **jojoba** is not available)

or

5 drops **sandalwood**
5 drops **bergamot**
in 10ml **jojoba** (This blend should not be used prior to going out in the sun.)

Niaouli cough mixture

1 drop **niaouli**
1 teaspoon clear honey
Mix well in a small bowl.
Small amounts of this mixture may be taken hourly for sore throats, ticklish coughs, and loss of voice.

Slimming oil

(massage oil)
13 drops **cypress**
12 drops **juniper**
in 50ml **jojoba**

or

2 drops **cypress**
2 drops **juniper**
in 2 teaspoons base oil

Indigestion remedy

1 drop **peppermint** oil
½ teaspoon honey
(or brown sugar)
½ cup hot water
Stir vigorously, and sip from the spoon.

Influenza rub

15 drops **lavender**
10ml base oil

or

2ml **ravansara**
100ml **camellia** (or other fatty base oil)
Rub into calves, upper arms, and wherever needed.

Mouthwash

1 drop **peppermint**
1 drop **lemon**
1 drop **clary sage**
in 100ml water

or

1 drop **rose**
1 drop **bergamot**
in 100ml water

or

1 drop **tea tree**
1 drop **lavender**
in 100ml water

or

1 drop **orange**
1 drop **lemon**
in 100ml water

Skin pigmentation

2 drops **lavender**
3 drops **niaouli**
1 drop **rose**
3 drops **sandalwood**
2 drops **tea tree**
5ml **rosehip seed** oil
in 25ml **camellia** oil

Environmental fragrance

2 drops **bergamot**
3 drops **lemon**
2 drops **geranium**
5 drops **clary sage**
1 drop **basil** or **rosemary**
in 100ml water. Pour 10–20ml into the receptacle of an aroma-lamp, above the candle.

or

Blend the essences in a small empty bottle, and use a few drops on a source of heat, as and when required.

or

To make a larger quantity just multiply each essence by the same figure. For example if you want 10 times as much concentrate of essences, use 20 drops **bergamot**, 30 drops **lemon**, 20 drops **geranium**, etc.

Recipes for Chapter Six

Immune system stimulant

(massage oil)
7 drops **tea tree**
7 drops **lavender**
7 drops **bergamot**
4 drops **sandalwood**
in 50ml base oil

or

1 drop **tea tree**
2 drops **lavender**
1 drop **bergamot**
1 drop **sandalwood**
in 2 teaspoons base oil

Niaouli cough mixture

1 drop **niaouli**
1 teaspoon clear honey
Mix well in a small dish, take small amounts at the first signs of a sore throat.

Mouthwash and gargle

1 drop **tea tree**
1 drop **niaouli**
1 drop **lemon**
in 100ml pure water.
(Shake well before use.)

Glandular tonic

(massage oil)
5 drops **tea tree**
5 drops **lavender**
10ml **jojoba**

Internal medication for candida

3 drops **niaouli**
3 drops **lemon**
on ½ teaspoon brown sugar
Dosage to be no more than twice per day for a maximum of three weeks. If any stomach upset is detected, then either reduce the amount of oils to 1 **niaouli** and 1 **lemon**, or cease taking the oils until the stomach is back to normal.
(See 'Precautionary Notes' on page 160).

Recipes for Chapter Seven

SKIN CARE

Night oil for normal/ dry skin

(massage oil)

2 drops **geranium**
10 drops **lavender**
5 drops **ylang-ylang**
8 drops **sandalwood**
in 50ml base oil

or

1 drop **geranium**
2 drops **lavender**
1 drop **ylang-ylang**
1 drop **sandalwood**
in 2 teaspoons base oil

or

5 drops **geranium**
16 drops **lavender**
4 drops **rosewood**
in 50ml base oil

or

1 drop **geranium**
3 drops **lavender**
1 drop **rosewood**
in 2 teaspoons base oil

Oil for acne/oily skin

(massage oil)

12 drops **cypress**
13 drops **lemon**
in 50ml base oil

or

2 drops **cypress**
2 drops **lemon**
1 drop **lavender**
in 2 teaspoons base oil

or

14 drops **bergamot**
5 drops **cypress**
6 drops **juniper**
in 50ml base oil

or

2 drops **bergamot**
1 drop **cypress**
1 drop **juniper**
in 2 teaspoons base oil

Oil for dry skin
(massage oil)
10 drops **sandalwood**
7 drops **geranium**
3 drops **rosewood**
5 drops **ylang-ylang**
in 50ml base oil

or

2 drops **sandalwood**
1 drop **geranium**
1 drop **rosewood**
1 drop **ylang-ylang**
in 2 teaspoons base oil

Oil for mature skin
(massage oil)
8 drops **frankincense**
14 drops **lavender**
3 drops **neroli**
in 50ml base oil

or

1 drop **frankincense**
2 drops **lavender**
in 1 teaspoon base oil

or

1 drop **frankincense**
1 drop **neroli**
in 1 teaspoon base oil

Skin Tonics – Floral Waters

Normal/dry skin
4 drops **geranium**
6 drops **lavender**
in 100ml water (preferably bottled spring water)
Place ingredients into a bottle, cap and shake vigorously. Shake before each use.

Greasy skin
6 drops **bergamot**
4 drops **lavender**
in 100ml water (preferably bottled spring water)

Miscellaneous Recipes

Rose body rub
20 drops **rose**
5ml **jojoba**
in 50ml base oil (5ml of it **jojoba**)

or

2 drops **rose**
in 5ml **jojoba**

Facial mask

1 heaped tablespoon kaolin or fuller's earth powder
2 tablespoons water
½ teaspoon clear honey
1 drop **lavender**
1 drop **geranium**

Neroli compress

1 drop **neroli**
500ml water
Thoroughly mix together ingredients in a bowl. Soak strips of absorbent material (such as lint), or a face flannel, in the liquid. Squeeze out excess and place the cloth on your face. (Ideally the cloth should have a hole cut out for your nose.)

Hair Care

Treatment for greasy hair

12 drops **bergamot**
13 drops **lavender**
5ml **jojoba**
in 45ml base oil

or

2 drops **bergamot**
2 drops **lavender**
few drops **jojoba**
in 2-3 teaspoons base oil

or

10 drops **lemon**
5 drops **ylang-ylang**
10 drops **orange**
10ml **jojoba**
in 40ml base oil

Treatment for dandruff

10 drops **eucalyptus**
15 drops **rosemary**
5ml **jojoba**
in 45ml base oil

or

1 drop **eucalyptus**
2 drops **rosemary**
few drops **jojoba**
on 2-3 teaspoons base oil

or

25 drops **tea tree**
10ml **jojoba**

or

2 drops **lemon**
1 drop **ylang-ylang**
1 drop **orange**
few drops **jojoba**
in 2-3 teaspoons base oil

Treatment for head lice

25 drops **rosemary**
12 drops **eucalyptus**
13 drops **geranium**
25 drops **lavender**
in 75ml base oil

Treatment for hair damaged by bleaching/perming

15 drops **rosewood**
5 drops **geranium**
5 drops **sandalwood**
5 drops **lavender**
10ml **jojoba**
in 45ml base oil

or

2 drops **rosewood**
1 drop **geranium**
1 drop **sandalwood**
1 drop **lavender**
few drops **jojoba**
in 2-3 teaspoons base oil

or

15 drops **lavender**
5 drops **myrtle**
5 drops **geranium**
10ml **jojoba**
in 45ml base oil

or

3 drops **lavender**
1 drop **myrtle**
1 drop **geranium**
in 2-3 teaspoons **jojoba**

HAIR RINSES

Dark hair

2 drops **rosemary**
1 drop **rosewood**
1 drop **geranium**
in 1 litre water

Fair hair

2 drops **camomile**
1 drop **lemon**

To a 1 litre bottle of water, add the drops of essence. Cap and shake well. Essential oils do not dissolve in water, but shaking vigorously will disperse them sufficiently. Shake again prior to pouring the lotion through the hair.

Recipes for Chapter Eight

Relaxing back massage

12 drops **bergamot**
4 drops **geranium**
9 drops **sandalwood**
in 50ml base oil
or
3 drops **bergamot**
1 drop **geranium**
2 drops **sandalwood**
in 2-3 teaspoons base oil
or
12 drops **myrtle**
4 drops **ylang-ylang**
9 drops **lavender**
in 50ml base oil
or
3 drops **myrtle**
1 drop **ylang-ylang**
2 drops **lavender**
in 2-3 teaspoons base oil

Labour

(massage oil)
14 drops **clary sage**
5 drops **rose**
6 drops **ylang-ylang**
in 50ml base oil
or
2 drops **clary sage**
1 drop **rose**
1 drop **ylang-ylang**
in 2-3 teaspoons base oil
or
4 drops **clary sage**
in 2-3 teaspoons base oil

Stretch marks

(massage oil)
20 drops **lavender**
5 drops **neroli** (optional)
in 50ml wheatgerm oil
or
4 drops **lavender**
1 drop **neroli**
in 2-3 teaspoons wheatgerm oil

Constipation

(massage oil)
20 drops **marjoram**
5 drops **rose**
in 50ml base oil
or
4 drops **marjoram**
1 drop **rose**
in 2-3 teaspoons base oil

Antiseptic

(room freshener)
6 drops **bergamot** or **lavender**
in 500ml hot water
Several essential oils are antiseptic and the choice of essence will depend on which fragrances are well accepted by the pregnant woman. Choose from any of the following: **bergamot, lavender, myrtle, clary sage, lemon, orange, geranium, niaouli, eucalyptus, orange blossom, rose, rosemary, rosewood.**

Recipes for Chapter Nine

Healing the perineum

(sitz bath)
2 drops **cypress**
3 drops **lavender**
in a bowl of warm water

Sore nipples

(massage oil)
1 drop **rose**
in 20ml **sweet almond** oil

Mastitis

(compress)
1 drop **geranium**
1 drop **lavender**
2 drops **rose**
in 500ml - 1 litre cold water
or
2-3 drops **rose**
in 500ml litre cold water
Mix well before dipping in a clean cloth and applying to affected breast.

Post partum massage

10 drops **bergamot**
10 drops **rosewood**
5 drops **orange**
in 50ml base oil

or

2 drops **bergamot**
1 drop **orange**
in 2 teaspoons base oil

or

2 drops **rosewood**
1 drop **orange**
in 2 teaspoons base oil

or

8 drops **lemongrass**
2 drops **orange**
5 drops **geranium**
in 50ml base oil

or

1 drop **lemongrass**
2 drops **orange**
1 drop **geranium**
in 2-3 teaspoons base oil

Recipes for Chapter Ten

Head lice
(massage oil)
25 drops **rosemary**
12 drops **eucalyptus**
13 drops **geranium**
25 drops **lavender**
in 75ml base oil

Chicken pox
(lotion)
1 drop **peppermint**
1 litre of water
Add drop to water, cap and shake. Pour off half the contents. Refill with water. Cap and shake. Pour away half the contents. Refill with water. You are now left with ¼ drop oil to 1 litre of water.

Aching legs
(massage oil)
15 drops **lavender**
10 drops **rosemary**
in 50ml base oil

or

3 drops **lavender**
2 drops **rosemary**
in 2-3 teaspoons base oil

Niaouli cough mixture
1 drop **niaouli**
1 teaspoon clear honey
Mix thoroughly in a small dish, and give sufficient to cover the tip of a teaspoon. For sore throats and coughs.

Chest rub
(massage oil)
1 drop **lavender**
1 drop **tea tree**
1 drop **niaouli**
1 drop **sandalwood**
in 25ml **jojoba**
For rubbing into the chest when a child has a cough or other bronchial infection.

Children's bath
1 drop **geranium**
1 drop **orange**
mixed well in warm bath water

or

1 drop **lavender**
1 drop **clary sage**
mixed well in warm bath water

Tummy ache

(compress)

1 drop **camomile**
in 1 litre warm water. Mix thoroughly before immersing compress cloth.

Dry skin in infants

(massage oil)

1 drop **rose**
in 50ml **sweet almond** oil

Sinus rub

1 drop **inula**
5ml **jojoba** or **sweet almond** oil
A small amount should be spread across the sinuses.

Therapeutic air freshener

1 drop **bergamot**
1 drop **lemon**
1 drop **geranium**
1 drop **clary sage**
1 drop **basil**
in a bowl of hot water or other source of heat.
This combination of essences prevented an asthmatic from succumbing to an asthmatic attack.

Child's perfume

1 drop **geranium**
1 drop **orange**
in 15ml **jojoba**
The 'perfume' will bring harmony and light-heartedness.

or

1 drop **geranium**
1 drop **lavender**
in 15ml **jojoba**
This 'perfume' is soothing and calming.

or

1 drop **rosewood**
1 drop **clary sage**
in 15ml **jojoba**
This 'perfume' is uplifting, for when your child is upset prior to going to a party.
The 'perfume' can be made even more subtle by the addition of more **jojoba**. As well as smelling sweet and fresh, these perfumes will all be beneficial to your child's well-being

GLOSSARY OF METHODS OF TREATMENT

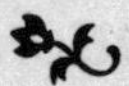

AIR FRESHENER/ENVIRONMENTAL FRAGRANCE

There are several ways to use essential oils as environmental enhancing air fresheners.

- Add a few drops of essence to a bowl of hot water.
- Sprinkle a few drops onto a carpet.
- Use a specially designed 'aroma lamp' heated by means of a candle.
  Drop your favourite essences onto the radiator in your hall, to give your guests a welcoming aroma.
- Buy an electrically heated aromatherapy burner.
- Use an electrically operated 'diffuser' which sends the essential oil into the atmosphere, but without heating it.

COMPRESS

A piece of material soaked in water to which you have first added your essential oils. It will vary in size according to the area to be treated. A handkerchief is the correct size for a forehead compress for a headache; a cotton wool ball for an eye compress; a hand towel or face flannel for stomach compress, etc. The water may be either warm or cold, again depending on what you are treating.

Sitz Bath

Also known as a hip bath. A few inches of water in the bottom of an ordinary bath, or a plastic bowl kept specially for this purpose. Add the selected essences to the water and mix well before sitting down.

Douche

An enema pot or plastic douche, both available from chemists (or surgical appliance centres), is filled with warm water and essences, which should first be thoroughly mixed together. Used in the treatment of vaginal disorders.

Honey Water

The easiest way of taking oils internally. Put one teaspoon of honey into a glass or cup, add approximately 1 fl oz (30ml) of hot water and stir until the honey is dissolved. Add the essential oil, and stir again.

Taking the mixture in teaspoonful amounts is the pleasantest way of taking **peppermint** oil.

Inhalation

Steam vapour inhalations to which essential oils have been added are used for respiratory conditions. Add your chosen essences to a bowl of hot water. Some people prefer to cover their head with a towel whilst bending over the bowl and breathing in the aromatic vapour.

Massage Oil

A blend of essential oils and base oils, such as **sweet almond** and **wheatgerm** oil. Sometimes **jojoba** oil is added. The usual ratio of essential oils to base oil is 2:98. That is 2 per cent essential oil to 98 per cent base oil. Two per cent of essential oil would be approximately 40-50 drops (to 100ml base oil).

(Please note that throughout this book, when 'drops' are referred to they are drops from any bottle of essential oil commonly available in shops or by mail order. This should not be confused with drops from a laboratory pipette, which are much smaller.)

On a Pillow

When essential oils are used on a pillow, as in the case of **eucalyptus** for colds, the essence should be placed at the pillow's edge, so that it does not come into contact with the skin. To avoid staining the bed linen, only use the essences which are clear or light in colour.

Skin Rub Perfume

A delicately scented oil which can be rubbed into the entire body surface after bathing. The base could be **jojoba** or one of the nut oils.

Internal Medication

As an alternative to using honey water when taking oils internally, add the essence or essences to a half teaspoon of brown sugar. (The use of sugar in this way is even acceptable when treating candida.)

Footbaths

A bowl of water to which you have added your chosen essences. If you have very sensitive skin, footbaths are sometimes better than any other method of treatment.

Baths

To your normal temperature bath water, add a few drops of your chosen essential oil and agitate the water before stepping in.

PRECAUTIONARY NOTES

- Some ingredients of plants can be toxic and oils containing thuyone should only be used by qualified aromatherapists. Oils containing thuyone should **never** be used by pregnant women. **Sage** contains thuyone, but **clary sage** does not. **Clary sage** contains a large proportion of linalyl acetate (the same as **lavender**).
- A very powerful ingredient of some essential oils which should not be used on the skin is safrol. It is a skin irritant. Essences containing safrol are **cinnamon** and **clove**. However, **cinnamon** oil is prescribed, internally, by French doctors for treating influenza, and **clove** oil is excellent for gum abscesses.
- When using oils on children, always remember that their skin is very delicate. Only use those essences which have been widely researched and written about. Oils which I use regularly on my children are **lavender**, **geranium** and **rose**. To be absolutely sure that the essence is adequately dispersed, place the correct number of drops into a 500ml bottle of water. Shake thoroughly before adding to the bath water and mix again with your hand.
- When blending essential oils for home use, remember that the essences are very concentrated and very powerful. Just because a little is beneficial, do not think that a large amount would work better. Only tiny amounts should be used.
- Externally, too strong a mixture can cause irritation to the skin. This will be characterized by itching, and a hot sensation. If this should happen accidentally, then apply pure **olive** oil or

a similar fatty oil, and try to dilute and disperse the essential oil. Washing the area with water will probably not help.

- If essential oils are used internally, they should be used with respect and caution. Many aromatherapists would argue that they should never be taken internally, because many of the essences are very strong and could cause irritation of the stomach. I do not disagree with this viewpoint, but the facts have to be weighed up. In the 18 years that I have been taking essences orally (e.g. **peppermint** for indigestion) I have never come to any harm. On the contrary, I am far healthier than in my pre-aromatherapy days when I used doctors' prescriptions to cure my ailments, or bought over-the-counter drugs. However, I must point out that a few people who have taken large amounts of essential oils internally for a protracted period of time have experienced problems which have been as serious as the overuse of aspirin or paracetamol. Thankfully these are extremely rare occurrences. If you are in any doubt, please consult a qualified medical practitioner or aromatherapist.

If we look to allopathic medicine we will find horrendous statistics of patients who have died or been damaged by the use of chemical drugs. More people in the UK, die each year from taking prescribed drugs than die in road accidents. More babies die each year from SIDS (cot death) than the total number of deaths which have occurred from AIDS since its discovery in 1985 until the present time. Experts in the field are admitting that there could be a link between drugs taken by the mother during childbirth and immediately after the birth, and some of the cot deaths. We only have to look at the Thalidomide situation, and compare that method of combating nausea to that of taking a drop of **peppermint** oil, to see quite clearly which form of medicine is the safer.

I could go on, but I am only expressing my personal preferences in the matter of taking essential oils. In France, essential oils are hardly ever used in the form of massage, as is most common in the UK and USA. Instead, the French doctors, who have taken a post-graduate training in aromatherapy, prescribe the oils for internal use, and have achieved great success with treating both acute life-threatening illnesses and chronic health problems. It is a matter for personal choice. There are a handful of essences which I use internally, but a great deal more than I only ever use externally, and as an intelligent adult, that choice is one I value and cherish. I exercise that choice consciously, and with confidence that the medicine I am using has been around for a long time, is well documented, and when used sensibly, is non-hazardous. And in that choice, I feel a great sense of pride in the morality of using medicines from plants. How many GPs can look to their consciences and say the same of the drugs which they prescribe? It is a sad fact that drug companies spend approximately £50,000 per doctor per year in persuading them to prescribe their drugs. Sometimes drugs reach the marketplace which are injurious to health, and have to be withdrawn from sale - it may be a few months or it may be several years after the initial launch - and what irreparable harm has been caused in the meantime?

We should also remember the enormous suffering inflicted on laboratory animals in the desperate search by the drug companies to find a 'best-selling drug', thereby increasing their profits and keeping the shareholders happy. Essential oils, although tested on rats for toxicity levels (the LD50 test), were tested more than 50 years ago and do not need to be re-tested. By employing essential oils as a safe and infinitely more pleasant alternative to taking prescription and over-the-counter drugs, we also, in an individual way, lessen the demand for chemical drugs. Hopefully this will, in the course of time, mean a lessening in the numbers of animals tortured and slaughtered in the name of medicine.

Some Useful Conversions

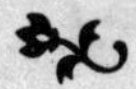

1ml = 20 drops
5ml = 1 teaspoonful
10ml = 2 teaspoonsful

2–3 drops of essential oil is adequate for 1–2 teaspoonsful of base oil
3–5 drops of essential oil is adequate for 2–3 teaspoonsful of base oil

Botanical Names of Essences

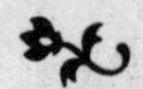

basil	Ocimum basilicum
bergamot	Citrus bergamia
camomile, Roman	Anthemis nobilis
clary sage	Salvia sclarea
clove	Eugenia caryophyllum
cypress	Cupressus sempervirens
eucalyptus	Eucalyptus globulus
frankincense	Boswellia carterii
garlic	Allium sativum
geranium	Pelargonium graveolens/ Pelargonium roseum
grapefruit	Citrus paradisi
inula	Inula graveolens
jasmine	Jasminum grandiflorum
jojoba	Simmondsia chinensis (Simmondsia californica)
juniper	Juniperus communis
lavender	Lavandula angustifolia
lemon	Citrus limonum
lemongrass	Andropogan citratus/ Cymbopogon citratus
marjoram (Spanish)	Thymus mastichina
myrtle	Myrtus communis
niaouli	Melaleuca viridiflora
orange	Citrus auranthium (fruit)
orange blossom (neroli)	Citrus auranthium (flowers)
peppermint	Mentha piperata
ravansara	Ravansara aromatica

rose	Rosa centifolia/ Rosa damascena
rosehip seed	Rosa rubijinosa
rosemary	Rosmarinus officinalis
rosewood	Aniba parviflora
sandalwood	Santalum album
tea tree	Melaleuca alternifolia
ylang-ylang	Canangium odoratum

BIBLIOGRAPHY

The Practice of Aromatherapy
Dr Jean Valnet (C. W. Daniel, 1982)
Primal Health
Michel Odent (Century Paperbacks, 1987)
You Can Heal Your Life
Louise Hay (Eden Grove Editions, 1988)
Unlimited Power
Anthony Robbins (Simon and Schuster, 1987)
The Family Guide to Homoeopathy
Dr Andrew Lockie (Hamlyn, 1990)
Vaccination and Immunization
Leon Chaitow (C. W. Daniel, 1987)
Maximum Immunity
Michael A Weiner, PhD. (Gateway Books, 1986)
What Doctors Don't Tell You
(a monthly publication available from 4 Wallace Road, London N1 2PG)

The Society of Homoeopaths has a free leaflet entitled 'Vaccination - A Difficult Decision', write to them at 2 Artizan Road, Northampton, NN1 4HU.

USEFUL ADDRESSES

Edward Bach Centre, Mount Vernon, Sotwell, Wallingford, Oxfordshire.

British Herbal Medicine Association, PO Box 304, Bournemouth, BH7 6JZ.

Institute for Optimum Nutrition, 5 Jerdan Place, London SW6 1BE. (Tel: 071 385 7984).

International Federation of Aromatherapists (IFA), Stanferd House, 2-4 Chiswick High Road, London W4 1PH. (Tel: 0181 742 2605).

Department of Continuing Education, Royal Masonic Hospital, Ravenscourt Park, London W6 0TN.

McTimony Chiropractic, The Institute of Pure Chiropractic, PO Box 127, Oxford OX1 1HH.

The Society of Homoeopaths, 2 Artizan Road, Northampton, NN1 4HU. (Tel: 0604 21400) for leaflet entitled, 'Vaccination - A Difficult Decision'.

There are too many different 'alternative' therapies to list them all. If there is a particular organization you wish to contact, either ring or write to:

Institute for Complementary Medicine, 21 Portland Place, London W1 (Tel: 071 636 9543).

USA

Essential oils from:

Scents of Smell, P.O. Box 7556, Boulder, CO 80302.

INDEX

Many essential oils are available through high street stores, but if you have difficulty in obtaining a particular oil or you are not satisfied with the quality you are able to obtain, please write enclosing a stamped addressed envelope to:

Maggie Tisserand
8 Paston Place
Brighton
East Sussex BN2 1HA

Tel: 0273 693622
Fax: 0273 676677

Owing to the sheer number of letters received, Maggie regrets that she is unable to enter into personal correspondence.

Always in stock:

- A large range of **pure essential oils**
- Ready blended oils of **rose, jasmine, neroli, inula**
- **Base oils** for face and body massage
- **Camellia oil**
- **Rosehip seed oil**
- Empty **bottles**
- Massage **bowls**
- Electric **fragrancers**
- Storage **boxes**
- Other **useful** products
- And how to obtain further information on the **honey cap**.

Write or phone for mail order brochure.

By the same author . . .

AROMATHERAPY FOR LOVERS

How to use aromatic oils with massage and gentle touch for stimulating and sensual love-making

Aromatherapy for Lovers opens up a whole new world of sensual lovemaking for you and your partner, showing you how to make the act of love truly holistic: mentally, physically and emotionally.

Discover:

- How to make up sexy massage oils and 'love potions'
- how to soothe and relax your partner with touch and fragrance
- ideas for scented lingerie, pillows and sheets
- how to use finger pressure and trigger points to help with sexual difficulties
- oils for beautifying your skin and making it silky to the touch
- aromatic remedies for massaging onto delicate body parts

Full of practical techniques and inspiring ideas, this book will enhance your love life, excite your partner and bring out your hidden sensual depths.

0-7225-2762-4 £4.99